"Neurodivergent students are successfully getting into Colleges/Universities but struggle unnecessarily and unfairly, affecting their mental health significantly once they get here. Consultation with Ruth enables the therapists at Student Wellness Services to help neurodivergent students navigate a system that is not designed for them. Ruth's knowledge is global as well as granular, having come from her extensive body of acquired knowledge as well as working with many, many neurodivergent folx over the years. Its knowledge you can trust!"

Jo-ann Ferreira, *BSW, RSW, M.Ed. (Counselling Psychology),*
Clinical Manager, Student Wellness Services, Queen's University

"With *Neurodiversity-Affirming Psychotherapy* Ruth offers solid guidance for clinicians embracing the opportunity for a much-needed paradigm shift in clinical practice. Blending trauma-informed, relationship focused, and co-regulation strategies to affirm neurodivergent identities is the pathway to autistic mental health. Ruth's clinical expertise and accessible communication blend to provide an indispensable framework for neurodiversity-affirming clinical practice."

Tess Clifford, *Ph.D., C.Psych., Psychologist*

"Having experienced misdiagnosis and oversight of my neurodivergence by the mental health system, I recognize the importance of guides like this. By shedding light on the nuances of neurodiversity, Ruth's book, *Neurodiversity-Affirming Psychotherapy* equips psychotherapists with the necessary insights and strategies to recognize neurodivergence, provide affirming and effective support, and prevent others from enduring the unnecessary pain and misdirection I experienced in my youth."

Emily

W0114806

Neurodiversity-Affirming Psychotherapy

Neurodiversity-Affirming Psychotherapy: Clinical Pathways to Autistic Mental Health provides an attachment-based framework within which clinicians can support autistic/neurodivergent clients to benefit from effective, trauma-informed psychotherapy.

This book builds upon practice-based evidence to guide neurotypical psychotherapists in case conceptualization and treatment planning for autistic/neurodivergent individuals, many of whom received behaviour modification rather than psychotherapy to address mental health needs in childhood.

Widening the lens on autistic wellbeing, the author addresses multiple features of diagnosed and undiagnosed neurodivergence, highlighting the pivotal elements of communication, sensory processing, and executive functioning, and emphasizing secure attachment relationships as foundational to mental health. Throughout the book, the neurodiversity-affirming approach and framework are illuminated through clinical examples.

This book delivers practical guidance and clinical insight, offering therapists a clear understanding of the mental health issues commonly experienced by autistic/neurodivergent adults, and guiding them and their clients along a robust pathway to autistic mental health.

Ruth M. Strunz is a Registered Psychotherapist and Clinical Supervisor specializing in cross-neurotype attachment relationships, across the lifespan. Ruth's model of Neurodiversity-Affirming Psychotherapy is grounded in extensive practice-based evidence. She brings over 25 years of clinical experience to training and mentoring clinicians in neurodiversity-affirming psychotherapy, across Canada and internationally.

Neurodiversity-Affirming Psychotherapy

Clinical Pathways to Autistic Mental Health

Ruth M. Strunz

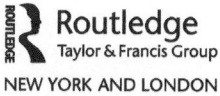

Routledge
Taylor & Francis Group

NEW YORK AND LONDON

Designed cover image: ©Getty Images

First published 2025
by Routledge
605 Third Avenue, New York, NY 10158

and by Routledge
4 Park Square, Milton Park, Abingdon, Oxon, OX14 4RN

Routledge is an imprint of the Taylor & Francis Group, an informa business

ISBN: 9781032553931 (hbk)
ISBN: 9781032553924 (pbk)
ISBN: 9781003430476 (ebk)

DOI: 10.4324/9781003430476

Typeset in Times New Roman
by Newgen Publishing UK

This book is dedicated to every autistic individual in my world.

You know who you are.

I am beyond grateful to you, and for you, always.

Contents

Preface

Neurodiversity-Affirming Psychotherapy has several specific goals. It provides guidance for neurotypical clinicians who want to work with autistic/neurodivergent clients and need additional competency to do so safely and effectively. It also invites reflective practice, supporting clinicians who are encountering difficulties in establishing or deepening a therapeutic alliance to reflect on what is happening in the space between themselves and the specific client; to become curious about whether they are navigating a cross-neurotype therapeutic alliance, and even to change course to safeguard the relationship. Thirdly, this book dips into the wonder of cross-neurotype attachment; I believe that humans are here to learn how to love one another, and I am fascinated by the ways that people with different neurotypes co-regulate within secure attachment relationships. And lastly, this book broaches some difficult questions, challenging neuronormativity in the dominant culture while eliciting the best in psychotherapists, within their intersecting roles as professional helpers, social justice advocates, and caring, compassionate human beings.

I started this book with a destination in mind, and a beautiful, hand-drawn map for how I intended to get there. Although I have arrived at that destination (or at least in the vicinity), the route has been extraordinarily different from the one I originally planned. Every forest path intersects with intriguing little side-trails, which a hiker may choose to take, or not. I have difficulty resisting exploring such trails, in forests and elsewhere. However, it is by leaving the main trail and following those little tracks that one comes upon those unexpected, quiet places that deepen understanding and widen perspective, opening space that was previously unavailable. I left and returned to the main trail many times while writing this book, and I do not regret those forays. As a psychotherapist, I am a listener and watcher, a holder of mirrors and keeper of stories. I am also one who follows the side trail, comes upon the view and gazes in amazement, releasing a long, slow exhale, and quietly marvelling at the wonder of it all.

It is true that we are a neurodiverse species, and therefore that neurotypical therapists need to know how to hold space for neurodivergent clients – at least until neurodivergence is appropriately represented in the population of coun-selling professionals. It is also true that I know some things about attachment-based therapies, and some things about autism/neurodivergence, and that I have a particular interest in and commitment to, easing human suffering. I am grateful for the many intersecting paths that have led me to writing his book, and equally grateful for whatever paths in your own life have led you to reading it.

Language is a powerful tool, with some sharp edges that must be used with care. In my role as a Clinical Supervisor, I encourage therapists to use the same language that their clients use to self-identify, even when it differs from their own preferred terminology. In my experience, shared language deepens the therapeutic alliance, and clinician inflexibility with language can result in therapeutic rupture. I also support clinicians to visit and reflect on the outer edges of their own comfort with terminology, thus expanding their capacity for social justice. In keeping with my own preference (and the preference of a great many neurodivergent individuals whom I admire) this book uses identity-first language; I use the terms "autistic individual" and "autistic person" throughout the text. I also use the blended term "autistic/neurodivergent", highlighting the interwoven threads of neurodivergence. Conversely, I do not use person-first terminology, such as "person with autism", because it promotes the implication that an individual and their autism can be separated from one another, which is neither true nor helpful! Additionally, while many neurodivergent individuals express comfort with it, I don't use the expression "on the autism spectrum" because it sounds to me like a fairground ride which one may climb on or off, as preferred. The bottom line is that in session with their therapist, the client gets to articulate their own identity (if not in psychotherapy, then where, truly?). In writing, the author gets to use the language that seems to best express their mes-sage. And in social justice, the advocate seeks to use language that will build the necessary bridges. Language, indeed, is a powerful device, in shaping human experience; I have endeavoured to use it carefully, mindfully, and fearlessly, within this book, just as I use it in session with my clients.

ADHD appears in this book in the context of a commonly co-occurring diag-nosis among autistic individuals. Allistic (non-autistic) people who have ADHD often identify as neurodivergent, and experience both the sensory processing and executive functioning aspects of neurodivergence. I identify as a neuro-divergent clinician and author. I have ADHD and therefore the completion of this book included exploring several irresistible forest trails – but the view was always worth it! There is significantly more information and support already available for clinicians who are working with clients with ADHD, and therefore I have oriented this book more toward those who support autistic individuals, diagnosed or otherwise. It is safe to say that many of the suggested strategies and supports will be helpful to folx who are neurodivergent and not autistic; in fact, they can safely be used to support any client who finds them helpful, for any reason.

I am a neurodivergent psychotherapist, a neurodivergent clinical supervisor, and a neurodivergent spouse and parent. And I am grateful to you, whatever your own neurotype, for walking a little of this path with me. My heartfelt hope is that it will pave the way for you to walk alongside your neurodivergent clients, with a neurodiversity-affirming abundance of heart, hope and happiness, on the journey.

Ruth M. Strunz
April, 2024

Acknowledgements

It is my daily practice to connect with gratitude, for my mental health and for my own delight. I highly recommend such reflective practices because they work. I also know that if I were to express gratitude to every individual who has contributed to this book, that list would fill a book by itself (and what a beautiful book it would be!).

As a psychotherapist, the people I want to thank most openly and abundantly for their contributions to this book – my clients – cannot be named. I can only say that if you have worked with me in psychotherapy, I am grateful to you, beyond all words, for your trust, your courage, your story, for every stone we have turned over together, and every moment we have shared. As an author, I am grateful to every clinician, every person, who reads this book; I needed to write it because you needed to read it. Therefore, you have given me a great gift, for which I will be forever grateful.

So many wonderful people have supported my work and encouraged my spirit, along this journey. To all those who have shared time and space with me, who have fed me, who have listened and challenged and shared and questioned, I am so grateful to you all. Particularly heartfelt gratitude to Julia Avery, Heather Berry, Christine Cho, Jenny Dungan, Fiona Coffey, Sandra Collins, Simon Gregory and Peter Kerrigan, Paul Jerry, Gord Langill, Evalyn and Suzie, Pam Smith, Cordula Wiegand, and Aviva Zukerman-Schure.

So much gratitude to my friend and mentor, Sandy Fiegehen, for creating a huge enough space for this book to materialize; and to my friend and colleague Susan King Gilchrist, for patience, organization, and intuition.

Boundless gratitude to my adult children, Sam, Oisin, and Genna; thank you to each of you for being exactly who are, and to all of you for snuggling down forever, in the heart of my heart.

Gratitude to Norah and Peter; I carry your precious lives, inside my own. Deepest gratitude to my brother Dave, for all the ways you support me. And gratitude to Lauren, Sawyer, and Haydn, for sharing your Dad with me, and for making me the Mum of six incredible adults!

An ocean of shining gratitude to my life partner, Stephan Flemming: thank you for your uncompromising belief in my work, and in the need for this book; for the breadth of your mind and the depth of your love; I am so grateful to be living our own, unique, happily-ever-after, with you.

And lastly, the pages of this book resonate with many autistic/neurodivergent voices; individuals I have not yet had the privilege of meeting in person. I centre these voices, in concert with the voices of my clients; their lived experience and significant contributions to the literature, are invaluable sources of learning for the mental health community. I respectfully express gratitude to these inspirational people, for all that you are and all that you do to lift neurodiversity into the light through your research, teaching, clinical work and your own neurodivergent persona, in the world: Laura Carravallah, Nicholas Chown, Mary Doherty, Mel Houser, Mona Johnson, Damian Milton, Megan Anna Neff, Stuart Neilson, Jane O'Sullivan, Devon Price, Claire-Eliza Sehinson, Sebastian Shaw, and Judy Singer.

Abbreviations and Acronyms

AASA   Adult and Adolescent Sensory Assessment
ACEs   Adverse Childhood Experiences
ABA   Applied Behaviour Analysis
ADD   Attention Deficit Disorder (terminology no longer in clinical use)
ADHD   Attention-Deficit Hyperactivity Disorder
ASD   Autism Spectrum Disorder
BPD   Borderline Personality Disorder
CAPD   Central Auditory Processing Disorder
DS   Down Syndrome
GFPP   Goal Focussed Positive Psychotherapy
HSP   Highly Sensitive Person
NAP   Neurodiversity-Affirming Psychotherapy
OCD   Obsessive Compulsive Disorder
PTSD   Post-Traumatic Stress Disorder
SID   Sensory Integration Disorder
SPD   Sensory Processing Disorder
SCD   Social Communication Disorder
SMART   Specific, Measurable, Attainable, Realistic, Time-bound
SUD   Substance Use Disorder
TS   Tourette Syndrome

Glossary

Ableism   Discriminatory or prejudicial treatment of people with disabilities based upon the assumption that typical abilities are superior or preferable.

Alexithymia   Difficulty in experiencing or expressing emotion.

Asperger's Syndrome/Autism Spectrum Disorder level 1   A neurological and developmental arrangement affecting how people interact, communicate, learn, and experience the world around them.

Attachment Relationship   A significant relationship involving exchange of care and comfort between humans.

Autistic Burnout   Intense psychological and physical exhaustion, sometimes experienced by autistic people in response to overload.

Behaviour Modification   A technique of operant conditioning intended to change, eliminate or stimulate specific behaviours.

Case Conceptualization   Gathering a client's presenting issues, history, patterns, and themes and interpreting them through the therapist's preferred theoretical framework, to guide treatment.

Cross-Cultural Competence   Ability to recognize, understand, and respond effectively to culturally based differences in values, beliefs and behaviours.

Cross-Neurotype Psychotherapy   Psychotherapy where the therapist and client have, or may have, different neurotypes from one another.

Dysregulation   Departure and difficulty returning to a state of inner equilibrium, temporarily, reducing access to the prefrontal cortex or thinking brain.

Executive Functioning   Higher-level cognitive processing including planning, initiating, coordinating, and conducting mental or physical activity.

Hyper-hyposensitivity   Over- or under-reactivity to one's sensory environment.

Masking   Intentional or unintentional strategies used to appear non-autistic in certain populations or situations.

Misophonia   Reduced tolerance to specific sounds, such as the sound of other people breathing, eating, filing nails etc.

Neurodivergent   Variation from typical neurological profile, with associated communication, sensory and executive functioning processing differences.

Neurodiversity   Umbrella term meaning the full spectrum of possible and actual neurological profiles in all human beings.

Neuronormativity   Societal perspective that neurodivergence is problematic, and that neurotypicality is the appropriate way to experience and interact with the world.

Neurotypical   Socio-cultural standard for typical or expected behaviour; opposite of neurodivergent.

Selective (or Situational) Mutism   An anxiety disorder in which a person becomes nonverbal in response to sensory overload or other increased or perceived demand.

Sensory Overload   A fight, fight or freeze response that occurs when one or more of the eight senses is required to process too much input

Sensory-Supportive Therapeutic Environment   Design of a therapeutic space characterized by accommodation of unique sensory needs to facilitate comfort and safety.

Therapeutic Alliance   The unique relational bond between a therapist and client, characterized by shared goals and an agreed-upon approach to pursuing them.

Trauma-Informed Care   A therapeutic approach that safely and competently addresses the client's trauma history as a pivotal element of recovery.

Treatment Plan   A clinically sound plan for healing designed by therapist and client, describing desired outcomes and identifying progress milestones.

Vicarious Trauma   Trauma symptoms experienced as a result of regular, indirect exposure to accounts of traumatic events.

Neurodiversity-Affirming Psychotherapy (NAP) and Applied Behaviour Analysis (ABA)

The contemporary dilemma

Introduction

It is axiomatic that people seeking improved mental health through psycho-therapy with a qualified clinician will, indeed must, engage in a therapeutic relationship grounded in mutual respect and animated by best practices offer-ing greatest opportunity for recovery and wellbeing. In keeping with the spirit and duty of the therapeutic profession, this book makes the case for adoption of Neurodiversity-Affirming Psychotherapy (NAP) as the primary therapeutic modality in autistic mental health, and disapproves the contemporary predom-inance of Applied Behaviour Analysis (ABA) in the care of autistic/neurodiver-gent individuals.

The book is organized in three sections. Early chapters review elements of the therapeutic process as practiced in NAP; middle chapters examine key aspects of autism/neurodivergence through the NAP lens; and the concluding material offers pragmatic guidance for clinicians choosing to employ NAP mental health-care with autistic clients. Throughout the material, every opportunity is taken to provide clear, practical mechanisms aiding in understanding and successful application of the NAP model. Non-identifying examples from my practice are provided where possible.

Chapter 1 responds to the following clinical questions:

1. What is *ABA*, and how is it used clinically, with autistic kids?
2. What mental health impacts of ABA are recognized and treated in NAP?
3. Where is the nexus among *Adverse Childhood Experiences (ACEs)*, autism, and ABA?

Overview – NAP: autistic mental health

NAP responds to the need for a clinically appropriate framework to guide and support neurotypical psychotherapists in working with autistic/neurodiver-gent adult clients. Autistic individuals encounter multiple barriers to accessing

DOI: 10.4324/9781003430476-1

effective mental health support, of which the most frequently reported is therapists' lack of understanding and expertise about autism, and related unwillingness to work with autistic individuals (Adams & Young, 2021; Lipinski et al., 2022). On the other side of the story, psychotherapists indicate that their training rarely addressed the mental health needs of autistic individuals, indicating awareness of this gap in their clinical competency, along with significant interest in receiving such training (Lipinski et al., 2022). Psychotherapists are generally highly motivated to help when they can and to do so both safely and competently, so it is reasonable to propose that an increased understanding of autism/neurodiversity will increase the neurotypical therapist's ability and openness to working with neurodivergent clients. One goal of NAP is to demystify cross-neurotype psychotherapy and increase capacity, by guiding neurotypical psychotherapists to develop clinical competency in working with individuals whose neurotype differs from their own.

My model for NAP is grounded in the literature on attachment theory and practice-based experience. This is natural and intentional, partly because I am an attachment-based psychotherapist, but also because one of the impacts of neuronormativity in healthcare is that autism is often described as a social or relational disability, or similar. It is appropriate therefore, to conceptualize NAP emerging in the nexus among attachment theory, clinical competency, neurodiversity, and social justice, wherever that place exists for you.

This book intends to educate, encourage, and support neurotypical therapists primarily, and to support their clients by extension. By highlighting the obstacles that autistic/neurodivergent adults encounter in accessing mental healthcare, it also demands social justice. There are multiple neurodiversity-affirming conversations happening in clinical, research and educational settings around the world, online and in person – find your people, listen carefully, and join the conversation! If you are in active clinical practice, it is more than likely that neurodivergence has already entered your therapy space, within or beyond your awareness. This book was written to help you welcome it warmly, hear it effectively, and respond to it with both confidence and compassion.

Consistent with the subject matter and my own neurotype, NAP was written in a non-linear, tapestry-like fashion. I recommend reading Chapters 1 to 3 in their entirety initially because they provide important context for what follows. The book can be read cover to cover if that is how your brain works best, and equally can be browsed and referenced as the need arises. You are invited to explore, discuss, and apply this material in whatever ways are aligned with your own neurotype and will help you to meet the mental health needs of your neurodivergent clients, safely and effectively.

Chapter 1 illuminates the unintended and unrecognized mental health outcomes of Applied Behaviour Analysis (ABA), a behaviour modification technique commonly misrepresented as psychotherapy for autistic children. The social justice role of the psychotherapist is addressed. For many therapists, this will be a challenging chapter to read. It was challenging to write, because it required revisiting a personal experience of vicarious trauma to recount a clinical anecdote which is as disturbing to me today as it was 13 years ago. This chapter includes voices from the literature and my own clinical practice, which will support the argument that although ABA can bring about behavioural change, when used to change the behaviour of an autistic child, it does so at an unacceptably high cost to the neurodivergent individual's mental health.

IMPORTANT: *This chapter contains a description of an actual ABA session with an autistic child, which was observed, filmed, and shared with me by his parent. It also contains the voices of autistic adults who received ABA in childhood. Clinicians and students who find this material disturbing are encouraged to explore their own responses further in clinical supervision.*

Chapter 2 introduces the concept of neurodiversity, outlines elements of diagnosed and undiagnosed neurodivergence, and describes the diagnostic features of autism spectrum disorder (ASD) and attention deficit hyperactivity disorder (ADHD). Chapter 3 guides neurotypical therapists toward establishing a therapeutic alliance with a client whose neurotype is different from their own and highlights a variety of common issues that autistic/neurodivergent clients present in psychotherapy. Chapter 4 discusses clinician selfcare, highlighting the interdependence of self-regulation and co-regulation as central elements of a cross-neurotype therapeutic alliance. Chapters 5 to 7 highlight and explore the three central foci in NAP: sensory processing, communication, and executive functioning. In Chapter 8 clinicians are provided with specific, clinically sound, practical strategies to facilitate NAP, some of which will resonate as familiar elements of familiar, evidence-based approaches. Chapter 9 discusses collaborative goal setting and monitoring progress with neurodivergent clients, and Chapter 10 focuses on attachment theory, while highlighting a variety of topics for further work, including clinician professional development, reflective practice, the neurodiversity-related needs of parents, and my nascent thoughts on neurodiversity-affirming clinical supervision. Prior to examining ABA, the available evidence on the current prevalence of ASD is briefly summarized.

Prevalence of autism

Reliable data on the number of autistic people (diagnosed and undiagnosed) in Canada, the United States, and United Kingdom are limited. Governmental and charitable agencies vary widely in how they classify, measure, and report on ASD. There is a broad consensus that the incidence of autism is rising across these countries among children and youth, but this view is complicated by increased diagnostic attention to autism in general, and to evolving understanding of how it presents among genders, suggesting significant under-reporting in the past. Recent dramatic increases in immigration across these countries, from populations with unknown autism concentrations, makes reliable estimation additionally challenging. Further, most sources seek to identify the number of people formally diagnosed, while recognizing an additional large but unknown proportion of undiagnosed autistic people within their borders.

Canadian statistics are particularly fraught. In the absence of well-defined and consistently collected incidence data and trend analyses over time (demonstrating the pressing need for this research is beyond the scope of this book), only broad evaluation is possible. The most oft-cited estimated proportion of autistic Canadians was reported by Anagnostou et al. (2014), positing that between 1% and 2% of the overall population are autistic. If accurate, and this proportion mirrors that found among other populations internationally in recent years, it is reasonable to conclude that in late 2023 the number of autistic Canadians was at minimum 405,284 and could be as many as 810,568.[1] Among this group, children and youth under 18 years across the country are estimated to total approximately 149,145.[2]

In the United States, the Centers for Disease Control (CDC) found that 2.21% of Americans 18 years of age and older in 2017 were autistic, totalling 5,437,988 people (Dietz et al. 2020). About 1 in 36 American children aged 8 years in 2020, or 2.8% of all children of that age, were found to be autistic (Maenner et al., 2023).

Data from the United Kingdom suggest relatively similar incidence. In 2018 the group diagnosed with autism (0.82%) plus those identifying as autistic, was estimated to total 1,197,300 people or 2.12% of the overall population (O'Nions et al., 2023). In the same study, the proportion of all children aged 10 to 14 years who were diagnosed autistic was much higher, at 2.94% or 1 in every 34.

Introduction to behaviour modification

Full disclosure is important: I am an attachment-based therapist, not a behavioural therapist. As such, I bring a basic understanding of behaviour modification to my clinical work, which can be helpful, specifically when supporting individuals (of any neurotype) whose therapeutic goals include making changes to their own behaviour. Identifying SMART (Specific, Measurable, Attainable, Realistic, Time-bound) goals (Bovend'Eerdt et al., 2009), and making desired behaviour change enhances quality of life, providing a sense of achievement and personal satisfaction for many people. In fact, like many therapists, I employ behaviour modification techniques myself when a personal tune-up is required!

The science supporting *behaviour modification* – generally described as utilizing basic scientific principles to change behaviour – is robust. Most adults engage in some form of personal behaviour modification sporadically, in pursuit of personally meaningful goals such as improving their own eating or sleeping habits, decluttering their home or work environment, or reducing their carbon footprint. There is nothing problematic, and lots that is beneficial, about intentionally changing one's own behaviour to better align with one's goals or core values, nor about doing so with the support of a trained clinician. If we don't like our own behaviour, or we believe it is causing problems for ourselves or others, intentionally and systematically modifying it is a reasonable thing to do.

However, there is a gap between using behaviour modification *to change one's own behaviour* and strive toward a personal goal – plant a garden or buy a bicycle – and using behaviour modification as a tool with which *to change the behaviour of another* person. That gap widens when the other person is a child and widens further when that child is in the pre-contemplative stage of change (Prochaska & DiClemente, 1982; Prochaska & Norcross, 2001) – unaware their behaviour is problematic and uninvested in changing it. However, the gap between using behaviour modification to change one's own behaviour and using it to change someone else's behaviour widens to a chasm, when the child's daily experience in the predominantly neurotypical world is mediated by the sensory, communication and executive functioning features of autism. Fundamentally, ABA is an operationalization of behaviour modification strategies that is used in clinical and educational settings to modify the behaviour of autistic/neurodivergent children.

They told me he needed ABA...

At her intake session, the young mother shared, with obvious sadness, the story of how her 8-year-old autistic son had stopped speaking during his last ABA session, the previous year. She described her little boy, who sang loudly while lining up cars and trucks as a toddler and enjoyed listening to her reading his favourite stories aloud, often filling in words at the end of familiar sentences with delight. Previously a chatty fellow with a sparkle in his eye, the child hadn't spoken above a whisper, nor uttered more than two words together, since the ABA session in question. Listening with one professional and one personal ear (my usual therapeutic stance) I heard a story I will never forget, despite my best efforts to do so.

The child's Grade 1 school report reflected that although he was progressing well academically, he had difficulty sharing classroom materials with peers, avoided group activities and withdrew from class discussions. At home, he had difficulty sleeping, definite aversions to certain foods, and often resisted leaving the house, even for outings that he would later enjoy. His parents requested assessment by a developmental pediatrician, who diagnosed autism and strongly recommended ABA to address his lagging social skills and atypical communication.

Some months later the child's ABA program began. The treatment plan involved initially working with an individual clinician on social communication, after which he would join a group of peers to practice his emerging social skills. His mother added that although the plan made sense to she and her partner, the start of ABA also marked the start of an endless stream of family conflict. Their son resisted going to sessions and developed "avoidance techniques" which included hiding under beds, encopresis (soiling his pants) and self-induced vomiting. When they managed to attend, his parents spent a torturous hour watching him through a one-way mirror, resisting a clinician (or two) who were intent on teaching him a variety of discrete social skills in which he had no interest. Frustrated beyond his tolerance, he regularly cried, lashed out at the clinicians, rolled around on the floor, or tried to leave the room. His mother described feeling waves of anxiety, self-doubt, and anger as she watched the sessions, often with tears running down her face.

The woman shared that she had filmed his last ABA session – the one at which he stopped speaking – and asked if she could show it to me. Hoping to gain some clinical insight into the situation (and never having seen an ABA session) I gladly accepted this opportunity. She located a video on her phone, and as she passed it to me I heard the sound of someone screaming. My vison focused upon a windowless room with a small table and three chairs (one lying on its side), on which a clipboard and some toys were visible. On the floor beside the table, a small child was writhing in all directions to free his body from the grip of two adults, screaming and sobbing as he struggled. For several minutes the dysregulated child thrashed his little body indiscriminately against the floor and walls, hitting and attempting to bite the clinicians who were restraining him. Eventually they forced him into a prone position, face on the floor, and used their strength and weight to hold him there. The little boy briefly resisted before he collapsed, face down and quietly sobbing on the floor, at which point they gradually released their hold from his body.

Deeply disturbed, I watched the child climb slowly to his feet and his mother entering the room, a panicked expression on her face. She hurried toward her son ... and then I saw the child turn away and withdraw into his own body, gaze lowered but vigilant, shoulders rounded, arms hanging loosely – filled with shame, and unable to trust the gestures of comfort that his mother was longing to provide. I rested the phone on my knee, and met the young mother's gaze, tears blurring my own vision. And then, very quietly, she said: "They told me he needed ABA, and I believed them. I let them do it and he knows that. If I was him, I wouldn't talk to me either."

Applied Behaviour Analysis – ABA

The neurodiversity paradigm appropriately recognizes autism as an identity, not an illness, and most psychotherapists would agree that while secure, stable identities may warrant personal exploration, they do not require treatment. Despite this, ABA continues to be administered widely as "treatment for autism", usually suggested to parents and caregivers by clinicians, immediately following a child's diagnosis.

ABA is a specific kind of behaviour modification that has been provided to autistic children since the 1960's. The approach uses *operant conditioning* to modify an individual's behaviour, using rewards/punishments to deliberately create an association between a specific behaviour and a positive or negative consequence (Staddon & Cerutti, 2003). Reframed as "positive and negative reinforcers", the rewards and punishments used in ABA include the provision of treats, withdrawal of privileges and withholding of valued personal belongings. The behavioural goals of ABA with autistic kids are generally intended to change the neurodivergent child's behaviour (including communication) to emulate more closely that of a neurotypical person. While ABA is promoted by researchers and clinicians, funded by governments, and actively sought by teachers and parents of autistic kids, it is simultaneously criticized vehemently by neurodivergent adults and allies, many of whom identify their own and others' experiences with ABA as significant causative factors in post-traumatic stress disorder (PTSD, see Kupferstein, 2018), intractable masking behaviours, social anxiety, and additional mental health difficulties. Acknowledging the humanizing changes that have gradually occurred in ABA since its inception, attuned psychotherapists hear the steadily increasing volume of autistic/neurodivergent voices, online as well as in clinical and academic settings, that reject this nominal "therapy" for autism, citing its adverse effect on mental health as an unacceptable (albeit unintentional) outcome.

Brief history of ABA

ABA was invented by American psychologist Ole Ivar Lovass (1927–2010), who also gained notoriety for his contribution of *conversion therapy* to the field of psychology; the parallel goals of the two interventions have not gone unnoticed (Conine et al., 2022). Conversion therapy with LGBTQ2S individuals is described as "any treatment, including individual talk therapy … which attempts to change an individual's sexual orientation from homosexual to heterosexual" (Drescher et al., 2016, p. 7). ABA with autistic children is described as

the use of operant conditioning (in which the desired behavior or increasingly closer approximations to it are followed by a reinforcing stimulus) individualized for the participant based upon analysis of observable behavior to make changes to behaviors that have been designated by the practitioner as abnormal or harmful.

(Williams, 2018, p. 67)

Viewed through the lens of attachment theory, both ABA and conversion therapy involve rejection of the self and experiences of betrayal by adults that the child/client most trusts to protect them, and upon whom they depend for nurturance. For obvious reasons, the provision of conversion therapy to LGBTQ2S individuals is now illegal in many jurisdictions, and for less obvious reasons, the provision of ABA to autistic children is not; rather it continues to be the treatment of choice, widely promoted by professionals in the fields of health and education, and hugely funded by governments and individuals across the Western world and beyond.

Certainly, science has demonstrated that ABA can change (modify) an autistic child's behaviour; with sufficient and consistent "reinforcement" in the form of rewards or punishments, almost any child will eventually produce the "desired" behaviour and/or eliminate the "undesired" behaviour. Collection of data is a significant element of ABA, and once the autistic child's changed behaviour enables the clinician or parent to collect enough data to demonstrate an "undesired" behaviour has been extinguished, or a "desired" behaviour has been established, the boxes are checked, the child's goal is met, and the treatment team feel successful. However, the cost to the child's mental health of trusted adults ignoring whatever they were trying to convey through behaviour, in favour of pursuing a goal that the practitioner or treatment plan prioritizes, remains unquantified. From a scientific perspective, that cost is merely collateral damage, but not so if you are that child, trading your sense of yourself and your own struggles, needs and opinions for stickers and candy, while gradually recognizing that nobody is listening.

The seeds of relational trauma

Fundamentally, behaviour modification of all kinds identifies and categorizes specific behaviours as desired, or undesired, and sets out to change/eliminate the undesired ones, while reinforcing the desired. Notwithstanding Kazdin's assertion that ABA is "not a bag of tricks, but a scientific approach to understanding and changing human behavior" (2013, p. 3), ABA practitioners are equipped with a set of techniques intended to reinforce desired behaviours and extinguish undesired behaviours in autistic/neurodivergent children who are immersed in emphatically neurotypical settings and contexts, without reprieve.

Young children of all neurotypes often express anxiety/discomfort through challenging behaviour rather than words, simply because it is more easily accessible – just as they may express excitement and delight by bouncing, dancing, or running in circles! Autistic children have varying degrees of language-based difficulties, increasing the need and likelihood of communicating-with-behaviour, especially in the early years. When parents, teachers and clinicians misinterpret challenging behaviour to indicate non-compliance or oppositionality, autistic kids understandably feel misunderstood, ignored, unsupported and eventually abandoned, by the adults they trust and love. The seeds of relational trauma are planted by repeated experiences of abandonment, especially in moments when the support of trusted adults feels critical to safety, or even survival.

Teaching neurotypical social skills to autistic kids

As described earlier, ABA is a domain of behavioural modification that largely uses *operant conditioning* to change behavior (Kazdin, 2013, p. 29). Skinner, 1953 defined operant behaviours as behaviour that has an impact on its environment, is emitted spontaneously, and is primarily controlled by its consequences. A commonly used example of operant behaviour is that of smiling; smiling is often spontaneous *in neurotypical individuals,* has a positive impact *on other neurotypical individuals,* and is often returned to the original smiler *by other neurotypical individuals.*

The process of ABA with autistic kids focusses on a specific, observable verbal or physical behaviour that is identified by parent or clinician as the target, either for elimination from or addition to, the child's behavioural repertoire. The behaviour is isolated and studied, with the intention of defining its observable antecedents and consequences, often referred to as ABCs (Antecedent, Behaviour, Consequence). Kazdin opines that ABA is "not about providing rewards for behavior" but rather is "about assessment, evaluation and intervention, and the integration of AB and Cs to change behavior" (2013, p. 11). Once the target behaviour is defined and the behavioural goal set, the treatment team (comprised of clinicians and parents) decides whether positive or negative reinforcers (rewards or punishments) will be most effective in achieving the desired outcome. Systematically, the adults use positive or negative reinforcers when the behaviour is presented (or suppressed) by the child and thereby an "undesired" behaviour is eliminated, or a "desired" behaviour is elicited. ABA is regularly employed with the goal of extinguishing so-called "autistic traits" such as echolalia, motor stereotypies, and sensory seeking/ avoidant behaviour in pre-school children (Williams, 2018). In elementary-aged kids, it is used to teach autistic children personal hygiene, self-care, and social communication based on the presupposition that these skills and behaviours will not emerge developmentally, even with appropriate, attachment-based support.

A range of behavioural reinforcers is employed by ABA practitioners working with autistic children. This may include positive reinforcers (rewards) such as stickers, candy, books, and even outings or experiences that the child enjoys. It may also include negative reinforcers (punishments) including water sprays or the use of contingent electric skin shock (CESS), effectively refuted by Fisher et al. (2023). Devastatingly from an attachment perspective, withdrawal of attention or affection by the parent/primary carer has also been used as a negative reinforcer in ABA. Within ABA programs, non-verbal or minimally verbal autistic children (in particular, but not exclusively) are physically and psychologically abused by adults, in ways that have long-ago been deemed unethical treatment of neurotypical children (Minshawi et al., 2014; Sandoval-Norton & Shkedy, 2019; Weiss, 2003). While we may wish that Kazdin (2013) was correct, the use of aversive techniques including physical restraint, isolation, withholding of basic needs and corporal punishment continues in many ABA-based clinics and schools – and it makes its presence known in therapy, when the therapist holds a big enough and brave enough space for the autistic/neurodivergent client to set down that heavy bag, and begin to unpack it.

ABA and secure attachment

Notwithstanding the persistent argument that ABA *must be a good thing because it is based in science* (a Western bias, indisputably!) one of the most significant problems lies precisely in this claim. The based-in-science argument has been used to support preposterous positions such as "Not all extreme beliefs about children with autism are negative … hopeful, positive misconceptions can be even more insidious, because they are often harder to discredit" (Handbook of ABA Intervention for Autism [Leaf et al. 2022, p. 38]). Such damaging worldviews are commonly held by scientists and clinicians in the business of behaviour modification for autistic children, effectively promoting the $17 billion ABA industry (Sandoval-Norton & Shkedy, 2019) while disregarding or silencing the voices of dissenting autistic/neurodivergent individuals and their allies.

ABA solidifies its science-based identity by highlighting that it addresses *observable* behaviour; however observable behaviour in people is determined by a blend of observable and unobservable criteria. While it is a relatively straightforward matter to train a child to say "please" to receive a desired reward on a good day – that same child's ability to perform the behaviour on demand may be compromised by unobservable factors such as emotional upset, sensory disturbances, physical discomfort, physiological needs, and similar. Continuing to expect or demand the desired "please" at such times places the child under unnecessary and unproductive stress. Additionally, autistic children navigate their day with communication-related obstacles, confusing or unreliable sensory experience, and executive functioning difficulties, often placing additional distance between themselves and the desired behaviour. It is no surprise then, that social skills – even those previously mastered – vary in autistic kids from day to day, causing frustration and disappointment within an ABA-influenced framework or environment. And, in a competitive and neuronormative culture, the impact on the parent-child relationship of repeated such "failures" is unlikely to be positive.

Autistic adults within my practice have identified various unintended negative outcomes of ABA in psychotherapy. These include a sense that their body is someone else's property, which evolved into significant body dysmorphia for the individual. Clients have reported social disempowerment, which they describe as debilitating anxiety around initiating interactions or joining groups; standing back and observing what other (neurotypical) people are doing before daring to suggest or initiate anything. Many children graduate from ABA with a pervasive pattern of prompt-dependency that consequently negatively impacts relationships (Bryan & Gast, 2000). Spouses of autistic individuals who received ABA in childhood reported that their partner's high level of prompt-dependency resulted in their feeling that they filled a parental rather than a partner role within the marriage (Wilson et al., 2014). Participants in the same study also disclosed that their autistic spouse's lack of motivation and need for prompting constituted a constant source of stress within the marital relationship (Wilson et al., 2014). By any standard, a clinical intervention known to carry such damaging side effects as loss of intrinsic motivation, pervasive self-doubt, body dysmorphia, selective (situational) mutism, prompt dependency, and even relational trauma/ insecure attachment, is highly questionable, suggesting that some ethical issues require serious examination.

Attachment theory and ABA

Case conceptualization in attachment-based therapy is informed by the client and therapist's exploration of the client's primary attachment relationships, which provides a framework for observing and reflecting upon subsequent relational patterns, whether problematic or beneficial. Although the therapist's specific clinical orientation will influence their interpretation and application of the findings of such an exploration, Burke, Danquah, and Barry (2016) observed that an understanding of attachment theory can enhance any therapeutic process. An exploration of early life relationships and their potential impacts on the client's relational behaviour and experiences thereafter is a comfortable fit with neurodiversity-affirming clinical practice.

Broadly speaking, attachment-based therapies recognize that an individual's patterns of relational behaviour reflect their relational experience with primary caregivers in infancy; secure primary attachment relationships are associated with increased chances of secure and satisfying relationships later in life (Crowell & Waters, 1994). However, life is a complicated journey, and relational waters may be muddied by various factors (of which neurodivergence can be one) and life experiences (of which an intervention intended to address the perceived deficits that have been erroneously associated with neurodivergence, may also be one). When an autistic adult seeks psychotherapy, and especially when they report relational difficulties, a gentle investigation of their attachment history is important. As challenging as the subject matter may be for therapists to raise, among autistic clients the possibility of relational trauma as an outcome of ABA, requires exploration, validation, and compassion.

The clinical delivery of ABA varies widely, but the underlying goal is always to *change the child's behaviour*. Irrespective of what a neurodivergent child may be trying to communicate with their behaviour, ABA sets out to isolate and extinguish behaviours that neurotypicals find challenging, and to replace them with behaviours that are more easily interpreted, accepted, or managed, in neuronormative social contexts. The mental health impacts of ABA treatment are typically described by autistic/neurodivergent individuals in therapy as "the price of fitting in" or similar. It is a costly endeavour, when the price-tag may include anxiety, depression, rage, low motivation, prompt-dependency, self-doubt, insecure/unstable identity, self-harm, suicidality, and/or selective (situational) mutism.

Adverse Childhood Experiences (ACEs) and ABA

When assessing a clients' relationship history in attachment-based psychotherapy, it is important to explore the relational impacts of intrusive healthcare experiences and prolonged or forced separation from primary attachment figures, in childhood. Through the lens of attachment theory, personal experiences in ABA described by autistic adults in my practice often align with the criteria for ACEs. Originally defined as exposure to emotional, physical, or sexual abuse, or household dysfunction during childhood (Felitti et al., 1998) this definition was expanded by Karatekin & Hill (2019) to include maltreatment, household dysfunction, community dysfunction, and peer dysfunction/property victimization. When the experience of targeted, systematic behavioural modification through operant conditioning in ABA regularly triggers a limbic response in an autistic child, relational trauma occurs. ABA was described to me by an autistic client as a "scary office where some kind of doctor gave me a sticker if I did what she wanted, and just sat and stared at me if I didn't." This autistic adolescent recalled ABA as a frightening experience involving perceived abandonment by their parents and forced compliance by a clinician (whose perfume always triggered a sickening headache, which lingered in memory long after the content of the lesson had been forgotten).

The impacts of ACEs on mental and physical health are cumulative; individuals who report four or more such experiences in childhood are at higher risk of health impacts (Hughes et al., 2017). This is important to recognize when working with neurodivergent clients, because autistic children are more likely to have multiple ACEs than their neurotypical peers (Dodds, 2021). Anda et al., 2008 confirm the dose-response relationship between client endorsement of ACEs and multiple psychological, and non-psychological, medical conditions.

This highlights the importance of exploring the neurodivergent client's recollection of ABA, and assessing how it was experienced by their childhood self. In my own practice, autistic adults have shared accounts of occasional or repeated incidents of forcible restraint, confinement, separation from parents/caregivers, and the use of positive and negative reinforcers they experienced, as confusing, erratic, and even physically painful. Some autistic adults have minimal detailed memory of their exposure to ABA, although they recall other childhood experiences with remarkable detail, raising the possibility of a dissociative response to a traumatic experience. Others have scattered, disjointed memories they intentionally suppress, uncomfortable somatic symptoms they ignore, frequent nightmares, and multiple other symptoms that would align with a diagnosis of PTSD, if assessed by a neurodiversity-affirming diagnostician.

It is understandable then, why many autistic people recall ABA in childhood as a profound and confusing experience of betrayal by adults, resulting in anger toward parents and mistrust of treatment providers. These individuals' earliest experience of "therapy" was painful enough to reasonably result in suspicion, fear, and staunch avoidance of any subsequent activity by that same name. Pearson, Rose, and Rees (2023) confirmed it was difficult for autistic/neurodivergent adults to establish a relationship with a therapist because they found therapists "difficult to trust, due to previous negative experiences." Ironically, since ABA treatment is administered in a child's formative years, its negative impacts are often so deeply engrained in the individual's belief system as to effectively preclude their access to the very help and support that is needed, and that NAP would provide.

Recovery and ABA

Therapeutic experiences that help clients find meaning and assign significance to their early life experience are central elements of attachment-based therapy. The recovery paradigm in mental health creates space for a personal journey toward wellbeing, as defined by each individual client in terms of their own experience (Davidson et al., 2005). There is a compelling need for clinical spaces that are intentionally accessible to autistic/neurodivergent individuals; sensory-friendly spaces where recovery from ABA or other sources of relational trauma is regarded as an essential and difficult conversation and framed accordingly. In clinical settings, the creation of neurodiversity-affirming physical and psychological spaces requires authentic concern, outside-the-box thinking, affirmative action, and sometimes deep courage. It is a wonderful thing to hear neurodiversity amplified by the voices of neurodivergent clinicians, researchers, educators, advocates, and influencers, navigating self-discovery, self-compassion, and self-disclosure. Every time those paths converge, as they inevitably do, truth is told, suffering is reduced, and somebody takes another step on the recovery journey.

A word to the ABA clinician

You are a brave soul indeed, to enter and explore this space – and you are warmly welcomed here. It is very difficult for professional helpers to examine the possibility, indeed likelihood, that even with the finest training and best of intentions, we will probably hurt some people more than we help them, through our work. Most of us are kind and compassionate people to begin with, and (without an external reinforcer in sight!) are highly motivated to help other people ease their own suffering. To our kindly natures we add a range of clinical competencies, blended with a mountain of experience and reflective practice, often requiring considerable personal investments of time, energy, and money. Our therapeutic bailiwick reflects our priorities and passions, our experiences, our interests, and our growing edges; all of which propel us in our work. We are also responsible to slow down and check ourselves, our clients and the landscape from time to time, to examine or challenge our beliefs and actions, and to hold ourselves and one another accountable for what we do, and how we do it.

There is excellent advice for professional helpers in the oft-quoted words of Maya Angelou (1928–2014): "Do the best you can until you know better. Then when you know better, do better." As therapists, if we believe secure attachment is foundational to mental health, it is essential that we courageously and compassionately reflect on our own clinical work through that lens. Our recognition of potential and recognized trauma experienced by autistic/neurodivergent kids in ABA, and our willingness to reflect, challenge and change whatever needs changing, is necessary. Therein lies the path to recovery of robust mental health for autistic/neurodivergent individuals who were hurt in ABA, restitution for ABA clinicians and their clients, and additional, sparkling grains of justice and mental wellbeing for us all to play in together, on the great sandy beach of the world.

They told me he needed ABA ... what he really needed was me

The story with which this chapter started, ended almost 2 years later. The relationship between the child and his mother clearly needed repair, but before we involved the child, the young woman agreed (somewhat reluctantly) to explore her own attachment history in therapy with me. That exploration allowed her to recognize how her childhood experiences in a military family had resulted in a relational pattern of deference to authority, leaving her vulnerable to feeling powerless and even silencing her, in response to perceived expertise. Our early work focused on recognizing how underlying beliefs from her childhood continued to influence her interpersonal relationships in adulthood. Her parenting style was thus influenced, as was her relationship with her beloved son. Grief and anger joined our sessions, as did courage, determination, and compassion; the mother's own recovery journey moved forward from there.

Two months after our initial meeting I prepared to meet her beautiful, quiet, autistic child. We met in a softly lit playroom, with a small number of toys and fidgets available, and his mom and I sat down and chatted quietly, while he explored the space. There was no pressure to interact, and no requirement to do anything – he was welcome to look at, listen to, touch, taste, or smell whatever caught his interest. Over several sessions, we conveyed non-verbally to the child that he was welcome in this space, that it would look and feel similar at each visit, and there was no demand on him to speak, be, or do anything while we were there together. His mom and I were available if he needed help to investigate something, but our central goal was to provide repeated experiences of co-regulation and unconditional acceptance, within a sensory environment tailored to his needs, much as a new parent does for an infant.

When it was clear he was entering the space easily and felt comfortable being there, his mom and I began to invite him to join our interactions, always in non-verbal ways. With continuous attention to our own self-regulation, we played slow, patterned games with balls or blocks, ensuring there were no sudden movements or loud sounds and there was always a space for him to join us. We welcomed him without fanfare when he did so; sometimes we just included him while the game continued. Gradually, we added small variations to our games – pauses for shared emotion, gradual increases in animation, momentary shifts away from the pattern and back to it – and over time the child's level of curiosity, emotional self-expression, and level of engagement with us deepened. On the day that he walked into the playroom, grabbed a brightly coloured ball, looked at me briefly and loudly announced "Mom's turn!" our work was essentially done.

Resilience in relationships requires secure attachment. Secure attachment requires unconditional acceptance, and unconditional acceptance means that individuals are seen and welcomed exactly as they are today, on an ongoing basis. No behavioural reinforcer will eliminate feelings of insecurity or fear, nor elicit love, trust, and connection. For those who recognize belonging as foundational to mental health, the "desired" behaviours and social skills that ABA can elicit in autistic kids are generally empty, meaningless demonstrations of compliance. The experience of unconditional acceptance, and the feelings of trust and connection, are the positive reinforcers that human beings need and from which they can learn. In the absence of these relational elements, nothing therapeutic is happening, in ABA or anywhere else.

Social justice

Many autistic/neurodivergent individuals experience discrimination in multiple contexts of their lives – often to the extent that they do not recognize it when it happens. From nursery school through elementary school, high school and university or college, autistic learners are excluded from learning opportunities that are inaccessible because of the sensory, communication and executive functioning features of autism. More accurately, these learning opportunities are inaccessible to autistic people because of neuronormativity, and ableism, and the unwillingness of decision-makers to recognize and respond to individual needs. Within my own clinical practice, I have joined parents in advocating for their autistic/neurodivergent kids to be included at school, included at camp, included at birthday parties – rather than excluded. I have advocated alongside autistic students for inclusive learning environments, inclusive grading structures and non-discriminatory disciplinary actions, and participated in advocacy initiatives in workplaces, universities and colleges, and in healthcare. Some real-life examples include:

- I have advocated for an autistic child whose teacher described her as "unfriendly, uncooperative, bossy, and controlling." The child was advanced in oral presentation and comprehension, but significantly behind her peers in basic math, and literacy ... she played alone at recess and sat alone at lunchtime, every day of her Grade 2 year. Neither the family doctor, nor the pediatrician, nor anybody at the school she had attended since kindergarten, had ever wondered whether she might be neurodivergent.
- I have responded to school board administrators who proposed during an Individual Education Plan (IEP) meeting that an autistic student should try harder to be nice, because there are "no resources available for an unfriendly kid who refuses to try."
- I have advocated with (and for) an autistic adolescent who was sexually assaulted by a peer at high school. School officials blamed the incident on the victim, citing their obvious academic ability and high intelligence as evidence of complicity.
- I have advocated for a neurodivergent student whose elementary school teachers chased and cornered him, lay on top of him to restrain him, yelled in his face, locked him into an isolation room, lied to him about the hidden presence of other staff... and then accused him of not trying hard enough to self-regulate.
- I have advocated with a pediatrician who asked, "at what point did a quirky kid become, you know, autistic?" (The answer was ... at about the same time his parents realized he had no same-age friends and preferred the company of adults; struggled with personal hygiene and basic grooming; talked extensively about certain subjects but never asked a question; never got invited to social gatherings; only ate six foods, all of which were beige or white; and knew significantly more about automatic garage doors than the technician who arrived to fix the one at home ... at about THAT point ...).

Effective psychotherapy does not happen in a vacuum, and its impacts are not confined to the therapy room. Psychotherapy is culturally situated, and culturally impactful. Regardless of the therapist's preferred modality or blend of approaches, psychotherapy supports people who are navigating hard and painful times in life. It increases coping capacity and decreases suffering, stimulates hope and positive expectation, and empowers people to make desired and intentional change. Effective psychotherapy also stimulates systemic change, challenges systems that cause suffering, offers appropriate alternatives, and supports positive social change. As therapists, we do this each time we discharge a client who has made progress toward the therapeutic outcome they desired. We do it each time we interact appropriately with colleagues, or other professionals. And we do it when we use our voices as tools for positive change beyond the therapy room, with and on behalf of our clients. Our abilities to take in and reflect on information, to attend to detail, to speak truth, to record stories – the same skills that make an effective therapist make a very effective advocate!

Advocacy that emerges from NAP will often include references to sensory processing and requests for communication adjustments, executive functioning supports, and adaptation of public spaces. Needs and requirements will differ among individuals, but clinicians are ideally positioned to empower autistic/neurodivergent clients to seek appropriate accommodation of their sensory, communication, and social/emotional needs.

As well as the clinical skills noted above, effective advocacy requires preparation, insight, courage, and determination. Like therapy, advocacy must be accessible, positive, and clear. Advocacy requires we understand who holds the power to make decisions in the setting and what are they bringing, both visibly and behind the scenes, to the table. Successful advocates know in advance what is needed and whom to ask, and they follow up after meetings, in writing. And autistic/neurodivergent individuals whose sensory, communication and executive functioning needs are attended to (by themselves and their therapist or other support person) make outstanding advocates!

Therapists have varying degrees of comfort and confidence in their advocacy abilities. Some enter the profession with experience behind them, enabling them to ask hard questions, to identify and confront discrimination, and to walk the path of resistance with their client. Not everyone has this background, but an understanding of social justice, and the willingness to speak out against injustice or oppression, is a clinical competency for psychotherapists, having met the fundamental, entry-to-practice requirements.

For some psychotherapists, life experience has honed the skillset needed for effective advocacy before entering training. For others the proverbial "fire in the belly" that fuels effective advocacy is kindled slowly, while listening with ears, mind, and heart to client's stories of injustice, discrimination, and oppression. Effective therapist-advocates are awake, alive, connected, and energized – they are not burned-out, struggling with vicarious trauma, nor are they typically counting the number of sleeps until the weekend! Self-care is as essential for advocacy as it is for therapy, and it is our professional responsibility to manage our time and circumstances, so we model mental health for clients. Only from this place of wellness can we fully engage with what is happening in the therapy room, and still have space and energy for advocacy, to address systemic problems at their roots. The Canadian Counselling and Psychotherapy Association (CCPA) Standards of Practice (CCPA, 2021) cite Toporek et al. (2005), positing that in the world of therapy/counselling, social justice involves "advocating for clients in their many social systems, modeling empowering behaviours by teaching clients how to access services, and encouraging clients to become advocates for themselves, within their communities." With ongoing client consent, effective advocacy stretches beyond the therapeutic setting and the clients' immediate community, to the wider society, and into the systems which purport to provide healthcare, education, and governance, in ways that are accessible to all. As clinicians, we are positioned to advocate WITH, and FOR, our clients. The decision as to which route is optimal in any given situation may be made by the client, with or without therapeutic involvement. In other words, it is the client's right to decide whether, when, how, how often, and with whom, advocacy is indicated. As with the many other hats we wear as psychotherapists, there is no avenue for client-related advocacy without ongoing and fully informed consent from the client.

While self-advocacy is usually the optimal starting point, an important discussion must occur between therapist and client if either has concerns that a discriminatory organizational culture may render self-advocacy unsafe. For example, in some school boards it is common practice to allocate 15 minutes for Identification, Placement, and Review Committee (IPRC) meetings, where students with special needs are assigned to a learning setting deemed by teachers and administrators to meet their learning needs, within the least restrictive environment. Parents are invited to attend the meeting at a specified time and place and are often simultaneously informed that the meeting will proceed in their absence and decisions will be taken whether they attend or not. The magnitude of this demand and its implications for their child is often overwhelming for autistic/neurodivergent parents, particularly when their own and the schools' perspectives of their child's needs differ. Most autistic parents are well-advised to bring an advocate to school meetings to support them in advocating for their child, but also to advocate for the parent in the moment, if communication becomes difficult in response to the demands of the situation.

It is reasonable to hope that the next generation of autistic children will be welcomed, valued, and unconditionally accepted – within their families, schools, workplaces, and the wider community. When this happens, the need for psychotherapists to advocate alongside autistic clients and their circles of care will be reduced. Neurotypicals will default to stances of curiosity, acceptance and understanding, creating safety for autistic/neurodivergent people to participate fully in public life, and to express themselves without fear of being ignored, criticized, or ridiculed. Public spaces and homes will be places of sensory support and refuge. Businesses will provide quiet hours, schools will genuinely value all kinds of minds, power will be redistributed appropriately ... and being autistic/neurodivergent will be recognized as a legitimate way of being in the world, rather than a stigmatizing mental health diagnosis.

Autistic/neurodivergent self-advocates often refer to the alienating experience of growing up and living in a "neurotypical world" (Mathur, 2021; Stockman, 2023), citing the environments they must navigate and the attitudes of professionals, systems, and the general population, as the most disabling elements of autism. Systemic advocacy for neurodiversity awareness and autistic mental health involves identifying and illuminating obstacles to fulsome participation in public life by autistic/neurodivergent individuals, suggesting accessible alternatives, and holding systems and administrators accountable for making necessary changes in attitudes, beliefs, physical settings, and behaviours. In the chapters that follow, a model for advancing the mental health of autistic/neurodivergent clients is presented, calling on clinicians to examine every aspect of their therapeutic practices in the light of neurodiversity, and to advocate for neurodiversity awareness far beyond the confines of their immediate clinical setting, and out into the world where change is so urgently needed.

Notes

1 Statistics Canada estimated the total extant population in October 2023 to be 40,528,396 (www150.statcan.gc.ca/n1/daily-quotidien/231219/dq231219c-eng.htm).
2 The United Nations reported that the proportion of Canada's under-18 population was 18.4% in 2022 (https://data.unicef.org/how-many/how-many-children-under-18-are-there-in-canada/). Applied to the Statistics Canada population tally of October 2023 (www150.statcan.gc.ca/n1/daily-quotidien/231219/dq231219c-eng.htm), there were 7,457,225 in that age group, of whom 2% may be estimated based upon the Canadian Health Survey on Children and Youth (CHSCY) to be diagnosed with autism (Public Health Agency of Canada, 2022).

References

Adams, D., & Young, K. (2021). A systematic review of the perceived barriers and facilitators to accessing psychological treatment for mental health problems in individuals on the autism spectrum. *Review Journal of Autism and Developmental Disorders, 8*(4), 436–453.

Anagnostou, E., Zwaigenbaum, L., Szatmari, P., Fombonne, E., Fernandez, B. A., Woodbury-Smith, M., Brian, J., Bryson, S., Smith, I. M., Drmic, I., Buchanan, J. A., Roberts, W., & Scherer, S. W. (2014). Autism spectrum disorder: Advances in evidence-based practice. *Canadian Medical Association Journal, 186*(7), 509–519.

Anda, R. F., Brown, D. W., Dube, S. R., Bremner, J. D., Felitti, V. J., & Giles, W. H. (2008). Adverse childhood experiences and chronic obstructive pulmonary disease in adults. *American Journal of Preventive Medicine, 34*(5), 396–403. https://doi.org/10.1016/J.AMEPRE.2008.02.002

Bovend'Eerdt, T. J., Botell, R. E., & Wade, D. T. (2009). Writing SMART rehabilitation goals and achieving goal attainment scaling: A practical guide. *Clinical Rehabilitation, 23*(4), 352–361.

Bryan, L. C., & Gast, D. L. (2000). Teaching on-task and on-schedule behaviors to high-functioning children with autism via picture activity schedules. *Journal of Autism and Developmental Disorders, 30*(6), 553–567. https://doi.org/10.1023/A:1005687310346

Burke, E., Danquah, A., & Berry, K. (2016). A qualitative exploration of the use of attachment theory in adult psychological therapy. *Clinical Psychology and Psychotherapy, 23*(2), 142–154. https://doi.org/10.1002/CPP.1943

Canadian Counselling and Psychotherapy Association. (2021). *Standards of practice* (6th ed.). CCPA.

Conine, D. E., Campau, S. C., & Petronelli, A. K. (2022). LGBTQ+ conversion therapy and applied behavior analysis: A call to action. *Journal of Applied Behavior Analysis, 55*(1), 6–18. https://doi.org/10.1002/JABA.876

Crowell, J. A., & Waters, E. (1994). Bowlby's theory grown up: The role of attachment in adult love relationships. *Psychological Inquiry, 5*(1), 31–34. https://doi.org/10.1207/S15327965PLI0501_4

Davidson, L., Sells, D., Songster, S., & O'Connell, M. (2005). Qualitative studies of recovery: What can we learn from the person? In R. O. Ralph & P. W. Corrigan (Eds.), *Recovery in Mental Illness: Broadening Our Understanding of Wellness* (pp. 147–170). American Psychological Association. https://doi.org/10.1037/10848-007

Dietz, P. M., Rose, C. E., McArthur, D., & Maenner, M. (2020). National and State estimates of adults with autism spectrum disorder. *Journal of Autism and Developmental Disorders, 50*(12), 4258–4266. https://doi.org/10.1007/s10803-020-04494-4

Dodds, R. L. (2021). An exploratory review of the associations between adverse experiences and autism. *Journal of Aggression, Maltreatment & Trauma, 30*(8), 1093–1112. https://doi.org/10.1080/10926771.2020.1783736

Drescher, J., Schwartz, A., Casoy, F., McIntosh, C. A., Hurley, B., Ashley, K., Barber, M., Goldenberg, D., Herbert, S. E., Lothwell, L. E., Mattson, M. R., McAfee, S. G., Pula, J., Rosario, V., & Tompkins, D. A. (2016). The growing regulation of conversion therapy. *Journal of Medical Regulation, 102*(2), 7. https://doi.org/10.30770/2572-1852-102.2.7

Felitti, V. J., Anda, R. F., Nordenberg, D., Williamson, D. F., Spitz, A. M., Edwards, V., Koss, M. P., & Marks, J. S. (1998). Relationship of childhood abuse and household dysfunction to many of the leading causes of death in adults: The adverse childhood experiences (ACE) study. *American Journal of Preventive Medicine, 14*(4), 245–258. https://doi.org/10.1016/S0749-3797(98)00017-8

Fisher, W. W., Greer, B. D., & Mitteer, D. R. (2023). Additional comments on the use of contingent electric skin shock. *Perspectives on Behavior Science, 46*(2), 339–348. https://doi.org/10.1007/S40614-023-00382-1

Hughes, K., Bellis, M. A., Hardcastle, K. A., Sethi, D., Butchart, A., Mikton, C., Jones, L., & Dunne, M. P. (2017). The effect of multiple adverse childhood experiences on health: A systematic review and meta-analysis. *The Lancet Public Health, 2*(8), 356–366.

Karatekin, C., & Hill, M. (2019). Expanding the original definition of Adverse Childhood Experiences (ACEs). *Journal of Child & Adolescent Trauma, 12*(3), 289. https://doi.org/10.1007/S40653-018-0237-5

Kazdin, A. E. (2013). *Behavior modification in applied settings* (7th ed.). Wadsworth/Thomson.

Kupferstein, H. (2018). Evidence of increased PTSD symptoms in autistics exposed to applied behavior analysis. *Advances in Autism, 4*(1), 19–29. https://doi.org/10.1108/AIA-08-2017-0016

Leaf, J., Cihon, J., Ferguson, J., & Weiss, M. (2022). *Handbook of applied behavior analysis intervention for autism: Integrating research into practice – Autism and child psychopathology series: Vol. eBook.* https://link.springer.com/content/pdf/10.1007/978-3-030-96478-8.pdf

Lipinski, S., Boegl, K., Blanke, E. S., Suenkel, U., & Dziobek, I. (2022). A blind spot in mental healthcare? Psychotherapists lack education and expertise for the support of adults on the autism spectrum. *Autism, 26*(6), 1509–1521.

Maenner, M. J., Warren, Z., Williams, A. R., & et al. (2023). Prevalence and characteristics of Autism Spectrum Disorder among children aged 8 years—autism and developmental disabilities monitoring network, 11 Sites, United States, 2020. *MMWR Surveillance Summaries: 2023, 72*(SS-2), 1–14.

Mathur, S. K. (2021). *Understanding the lived experiences of autistic adults*. Chapman University.

Minshawi, N. F., Hurwitz, S., Fodstad, J. C., Biebl, S., Morriss, D. H., & Mcdougle, C. J. (2014). The association between self-injurious behaviors and autism spectrum disorders. *Psychology Research and Behavior Management, 7*, 125–136. https://doi.org/10.2147/PRBM.S44635

O'Nions, E., Petersen, I., Buckman, J. E. J., Charlton, R., Cooper, C., & Corbett, A. (2023). Autism in England: Assessing underdiagnosis in a population-based cohort study of prospectively collected primary care data. *The Lancet Regional Health – EuropeEurope, 29,*, 100626.

Pearson, A., Rose, K., & Rees, J. (2023). 'I felt like I deserved it because I was autistic': Understanding the impact of interpersonal victimisation in the lives of autistic people. *Autism, 27*(2), 500–511.

Prochaska, J. O., & DiClemente, C. (1982). Trans-theoretical therapy-toward a more integrative model of change. *Psychotherapy: Theory, Research & Practice, 19*(3), 276–288. https://doi.org/10.1037/h0088437

Prochaska, J. O., & Norcross, J. C. (2001). Stages of change. *Psychotherapy, 38*(4), 443–448. https://doi.org/10.1037/0033-3204.38.4.443

Sandoval-Norton, A. H., & Shkedy, G. (2019). How much compliance is too much compliance: Is long-term ABA therapy abuse? *Cogent Psychology, 6*(1). https://doi.org/10.1080/23311908.2019.1641258

Skinner, B. F. (1953). *Science and human behavior*. Macmillan.

Staddon, J. E. R., & Cerutti, D. T. (2003). Operant conditioning. *Annual Review of Psychology, 54*(1), 115–144.

Stockman, J. (2023). *Notes for neuro navigators: The allies' quick-start guide to championing neurodivergent brains*. Jessica Kingsley Publishers.

Toporek, R. L., Gerstein, L., Fouad, N., Roysircar, G., & Israel, T. (2005). *Handbook for social justice in counseling psychology: Leadership, vision, and action*. Sage Publications.

Weiss, J. A. (2003). Self-injurious behaviours in autism: A literature review. *Journal on Developmental Disabilities, 9*(2), 127–144.

Williams, A. (2018). Autonomously autistic. *Canadian Journal of Disability Studies, 7*(2), 60–82. https://doi.org/10.15353/CJDS.V7I2.423

Wilson, B., Beamish, W., Hay, S., & Attwood, T. (2014). Prompt dependency beyond childhood: Adults with Asperger's syndrome and intimate relationships. *Journal of Relationships Research, 5*. https://doi.org/10.1017/JRR.2014.11

Chapter 2

Autism is a diagnosis – neurodivergence is an identity

The emergence and popular usage of the concept of neurodiversity has widened our cultural perspectives and understanding of the many different ways that individuals experience and interact with their environments, and the impacts these experiences have on their mental health. Recognizing undiagnosed as well as diagnosed (autism, ADHD, etc.) neurodivergence, therapists are called upon to widen their therapeutic lens accordingly, to ensure their skills and support is accessible to individuals of all neurotypes.

In this chapter, neurodivergence (an identity) and autism (a diagnosis) are differentiated, and the implications of that distinction are identified. The impact of ableism on autistic mental health is discussed, and a strengths-based framework for case conceptualization and treatment planning for neurodivergent clients is proposed, one that integrates the identity of the client with their medical diagnosis, as applicable. The DSM-5 (American Psychiatric Association, 2022) diagnostic criteria for Autism Spectrum Disorder (ASD, three levels) and ADHD (three types) are detailed. A shared understanding of the concepts of neurodiversity, neurodivergence, and neuronormativity and their appropriate usage is needed, prior to reading this chapter; please refer to the glossary.

Chapter 2 provides responses to the following clinical questions:

1. What does the term *neurodiversity* refer to?
2. Is every *neurodivergent* individual autistic? Does every autistic person identify as neurodivergent?
3. How can clinicians approach *case conceptualization* and *treatment planning* in neurodiversity-affirming ways?
4. What does the level of autism (in the diagnostic criteria) mean? What DSM-5 (APA, 2022) autistic profile was previously referred to as *Asperger's Syndrome,* in DSM-IV?
5. What is the nexus among autism, ADHD, and neurodivergence?

DOI: 10.4324/9781003430476-2

Neurodiversity, neurodivergence, and autism

Neurodivergence is a political term and may be a personal identity – it is not a medical diagnosis. Many (not all) autistic individuals value the inclusivity that is inherent in the values underlying the *neurodiversity movement* and gladly identify as neurodivergent. Concurrently, it is important to recognize that not every neurodivergent individual is autistic; people with many different diagnoses belong within the neurodivergent community. Additionally, any individual who self-identifies as neurodivergent also belongs within this profoundly inclusive community. Neurodiversity creates space for all kinds of minds, and many undiagnosed individuals self-identify as neurodivergent in adolescence or adulthood, reflecting their personal awareness that they frequently experience life quite differently from others in their family or community. Along with autism, a variety of clinical diagnoses are widely recognized as neurodivergent. These include ADHD, social (pragmatic) communication disorder, learning disabilities/differences (LD), including dyslexia, dyscalculia, dysgraphia, etc., central auditory processing disorder (CAPD), Tourette Syndrome (TS, motor & vocal tics), and Down Syndrome (DS, or trisomy 21).

The concept of neurodiversity was proposed in the late 1990's by Australian sociologist Judy Singer. Singer identified neurodiversity as an essential addition to the already-established categories of intersectionality that included gender, class, and race, among others. She also proposed that the civil rights movement for neurological minorities that she observed coalescing around the need for self-determination and self-advocacy needed a name; and the term neurodiversity captured the concept perfectly.[1]

Singer observed that within nature, ecosystems are interdependent, and that the greater the biodiversity within an eco-system, the more stable, adaptable, and sustainable the system. She extrapolated that the more that neurodiversity is respected and facilitated within a culture, the more stable, adaptable, and sustainable the culture will be. After interviewing her, political columnist John Harris quoted Singer's narrative around the birth of the term: "I knew what I was doing. 'Neuro' was a reference to the rise of neuroscience. 'Diversity' is a political term; it originated with the Black American civil rights movement. 'Biodiversity' is really a political term, too. As a word, 'neurodiversity' describes the whole of humanity. But the neurodiversity *movement* is a political movement for people who want their human rights." Harris appropriately acclaims neurodiversity as "the concept she [Singer] quietly introduced to the world in 1997."[2]

Identity, culture, intersectionality, and belonging

Identity – a coherent sense of who we truly are, across time and in all circumstances – is nestled in the bedrock of mental health. An individual's identity represents their innate, genetically determined traits blended with a set of values, ideas, and beliefs absorbed from their surroundings, and from those who influence them in childhood. Innate traits are generally static, but as humans grow, they have increasing opportunities to assess, keep, or change the acquired aspects of their identities. Making such change is sometimes complicated by reactions or resistance of other people who matter to the individual, or from systems that hold power within the culture. Erikson (1959) highlights adolescence as the life stage when individuals need to question their identities, accepting or rejecting elements of family and the wider culture that ascribed the social roles, values, and affiliations they absorbed in childhood. This need enables the adolescent to develop their identity based on their own values, which may be aligned with those of their family and culture, or not. Schmeck et al. (2013) posited that identity is shaped by social and cultural values, and by how other people (within the same culture) perceive and acknowledge one's innate, personal characteristics. This is important in reflecting on the cultural experience of neurodivergent individuals within neuronormative settings and systems that have emerged from neuronormative ideologies.

Culture can be defined as the shared beliefs, values, and behaviours of a group. Every individual within a culture brings their personal identity to the group; humans are social creatures, and the need to belong is a compelling motive for most. The sense of belonging with other people allows the individual to develop a cultural identity, although the cost of doing so may be as high as disguising or concealing innate aspects of their personal identity. Henley (2013, p. 18, as cited in Strunz, 2018) posited that "although we often take it for granted, our belonging with one another is the very stuff of life, equally important than [sic] the food and drink which nurtures us." Likewise, (Baumeister & Leary, 1995) observe that "much of what people do, is done in the service of belongingness." Attachment theory (Ainsworth et al., 1978; Bowlby, 1988; as cited in Strunz, 2018) recognizes infants' experience of belonging within their primary attachment relationship as their template for future relationships, and therefore as significantly predictive of their mental health in adulthood. From a mental health perspective, it appears that the life-sustaining human capacity for adaptation has a few strings attached, especially for those whose neurological arrangement is different from those who hold power in the mainstream culture. Somewhere in its collective psyche, spoken or unspoken, every culture has norms and expectations about ways of being and doing, to which those who belong, or wish to belong, are expected to conform. Inevitably, those who have difficulty doing so as a result of their neurotype will experience the impact of otherness on their mental health, sooner or later.

The theory of intersectionality acknowledges that people have multiple identities and are subject to intersecting forms of oppression (Crenshaw, 2013). Intersectionality is starkly applicable to the experience of autistic/neurodivergent individuals navigating daily life in a neuronormative culture. To feel a sense of belonging, neurodivergent individuals commonly disguise or "mask" core aspects of their identity. Viewed through the lens of intersectionality, masking in autism is a highly adaptive response to the sense of non-belonging that is familiar to many neurodivergent individuals from early childhood on.

Identity formation begins with a young child's experience of the interplay between their innate traits and their environment. Without the perspective that life experience offers, children see themselves essentially through the same lens through which their parents (primary attachment figures) see them. Kids who are loved and valued see themselves as loveable and valuable, and the reverse is also true. When the family culture reflects inclusive values such as curiosity, generosity, and kindness, a child's individual identity is likely to include acceptance and celebration of differences between their self and others. Conversely, kids whose family culture stresses conformity, conventionality, and unobtrusiveness are likely to form identities that emphasize fitting in, rule-following, and avoiding rocking the proverbial boat. For many individuals, the journey of identity formation, and reconstitution continues far beyond childhood, depending on internal wellbeing and external circumstances.

Identity-related questions arise as often as a therapist sees a client! Who am I and what do I value? What does it mean, to be who I am? Who am I according to my brother? My mother? My friends? Who am I according to me? Through the lens of intersectionality, these questions become more nuanced, and more interesting. Who am I through a racial lens? An educational lens? The lens of neurodiversity? Who was I then, and who am I NOW, according to me? A coherent sense of identity is associated with knowing one's values and aligning one's decisions and actions with them; having a sense of direction in life; feeling comfortable being oneself; feeling authentic; feeling safe. A coherent sense of one's identity clears the path to finding others whose identities are aligned, or unthreatened by, one's own. Psychotherapists are often privileged to walk a piece of the journey beside an individual who is seeking their true culture, their tribe, the people and settings that may elicit their own sense of belonging. This is a common theme in NAP because feelings of belonging arise when an individual is seen and valued as they are, and for who they are. However, the life experience of many autistic individuals differs significantly from this; realistically, the extent to which autistic/neurodivergent individuals need to mask to feel a sense of belonging, reflects the extent to which the culture in which the culture rejects and "others" their full, neurodivergent selves. Rogers (1959, p. 208) emphasized: "One of the potent elements in the [therapeutic] relationship is that the therapist prizes the whole person of the client." NAP is person-centred therapy, and the notable emphasis placed on the therapist's role in establishing and sustaining the therapeutic alliance above all else, is intentional.

Some diagnosed autistic individuals benefit from exploring in therapy the meanings they or others have attached to their diagnosis, and the impacts of those meanings on their lives and identities. Commonly, the theme of being different (or feeling different) comes up, accompanied by the emotions associated with the experience of isolation or exclusion by family or peers. When a childhood diagnosis of autism is associated with recognition, acceptance, and belonging, the groundwork for the child's positive self-concept is laid. Conversely, when the messaging conveys anxiety or rejection, the child's self-concept will reflect that instead. Autistic kids who grow up in settings that inadvertently (or overtly) convey that they are different from others in negative or challenging ways, or that their struggles or inability to conform suggests they don't fully belong, are subject to relational trauma, even in relationship with loving parents and caregivers.

With devastating frequency, autistic adults with poor mental health describe the childhood messaging they received from family, school or community was some variation of: *YOU belong, but your AUTISM does not*. Conditional acceptance has a profoundly damaging impact on the autistic child's emerging self-concept and personal identity, as they wade through the mud of neuronormativity toward adulthood. The messaging of neurodiversity differs significantly, with the associated positive outcomes in terms of self-concept and personal identity, and therefore on mental health. Kids who grow up in neurodiversity-affirming families and environments receive clear messages that: *You are autistic AND you belong* (not despite being different, but *because* you are different!). This kind of messaging supports positive self-conceptualization and facilitates coherent identity formation and self-acceptance. This is the messaging that NAP offers autistic/neurodivergent clients, gently and persistently engaging them in a safe, well-informed, co-regulated therapeutic relationship.

Common themes in neurodivergence

Neurodivergent individuals (with or without diagnoses) report regular and repetitive stress and experiences of overwhelm, highlighting their predisposition to mental health difficulties. When providing psychotherapy to neurodivergent individuals, it is important to consider the combined impacts of neuronormativity in dominant culture upon the common features of neurodivergence. Of note, many neurodivergent clients report that the following common features of neurodivergence, which are explored later in this book, have significantly less impact upon their mental health when they are out in nature, engaged in creative or artistic pursuits, immersed in their personal interest, or working at their own pace within a neurodiversity-affirming environment. With that, the following domains are often identified by neurodivergent individuals and their loved ones as areas of difficulty in career or social settings, and important relationships:

1. Sensory processing
2. Executive functioning
3. Communication

Alongside awareness of these three central domains, recognizing the damaging early life experiences that many autistic (and other neurodivergent) adults bring to psychotherapy, the importance of consistently holding a stance of unconditional positive regard (Rogers, 1959) cannot be overstated. In NAP, it is this stance, together with awareness of the common features of neurodivergence as outlined above, that facilitates change, allowing neurodivergent clients to acknowledge and accept their experience, bringing a sense of wholeness or congruity, and enabling them to function effectively in their own lives (Rogers, 1959, p. 208). The opportunity for an autistic/neurodivergent client to develop self-acceptance is largely dependent on the psychotherapist providing a neurodiversity-affirming therapeutic experience, which is necessarily grounded in unconditional positive regard.

Ableism and neurodiversity

In the context of autism, understanding ableism requires briefly visiting the question of (dis)ability. There is a wide range of opinions among autistic/neurodivergent individuals (and their loved ones) about the extent to which they are or are not disabled, within the social contexts of the dominant culture. An element of this question relates to the level at which autism is diagnosed. An individual with a diagnosis of autism at level three, may experience more obstacles to thriving, more often, than an individual diagnosed at level one – depending upon their own wellbeing on a given day, the task ahead, their own and others' expectations, and the supports or accommodations needed and available. Clearly, there is a subjective element to the experience of ability/disability, in autism. Many parents of autistic children identify commonalities between their kids' experiences and their family life with those of kids with more apparent disabilities, and many others note exactly the opposite. Perspectives, expectations, and experience show up here, as does the question of the parents' own neurotype and degrees of self-awareness. Autistic/neurodivergent parents who are thriving in their own lives are less likely to view their child's autism as a disability, than neurotypical parents who are navigating life with generalized anxiety, or a substance use disorder. In NAP, it is important to simply note that the language of disability works for some autistic/neurodivergent individuals, and for others not at all. In contrast, the language of ableism works for nobody.

Ableism may be understood as a system of discrimination based on the belief that typical abilities are superior to atypical. Societally, it manifests in overt and covert ways but in the world of autism, ableism provides space and voice for neuronormativity to persist. Neurodiversity refutes ableism, by recognizing that each person has a unique neurological profile, and that none are superior or inferior to another. However, neurological profiles are invisible, and people form opinions quickly, often based upon assumptions and superficial observation.

Consequently, autistic people frequently encounter ableism within the dominant culture. Ableism occurs when an autistic individual discloses their neurodivergence and receives a disbelieving or dismissive response; a microaggression. Similarly, ableism occurs when public settings do not provide sensory accommodations such as dimmed lighting or reduced sound, and when autistic people are obliged to endure unwanted social touch. Many neurodivergent individuals identify unrequested advocacy as ableist, occurring when other people speak on their behalf without their request to do so. Additionally, Bottema-Beutel et al. (2021) highlighted that ableism *within the literature* influences how people talk about and perceive autism, whether they are aware of it or not, and irrespective of whether they believe that autistic people are inferior to non-autistic people. They call on researchers and authors to rebut ableism by intentionally using neurodiversity-affirming language in all clinical and professional writing about autism.

The neurodiversity movement underscores that when autistic/neurodivergent individuals feel disabled it can often be attributed to the environment they are in, or to neuronormative expectations or demands embedded within systems, or to inadequate supports to navigate such systems. A familiar example is the inaccessibility of mainstream grocery stores to many neurodivergent individuals; the combination of the sensory experience (sounds, lights, smells) and executive functioning challenges (store layout, items moved around, decision-making, confusing signage, transit or parking issues) and communication demands (asking for help to locate items, navigating unplanned and undesired social interactions) makes grocery shopping an exhausting and demanding activity for many autistic individuals. Consequently, many autistic people shop late at night or on days when they have nothing else to attend to; some autistic individuals avoid shopping altogether by growing their own food, incurring the expense of delivery services, or making creative arrangements with friends or family members to stock the pantry.

Autistic advocates often highlight that they feel disabled in some contexts and not in others, and on some days but not every day, casting light on disability as a social construct. From a psychotherapeutic perspective, the question of whether an autistic/neurodivergent individual is disabled or not is moot; only the individual knows the answer to that question. If that individual is your client, ask them!

Strengths-based psychotherapy

The overarching goal of psychodynamic psychotherapy is to help clients gain insight into how they feel and think, and to explore how their past experience influences their present behaviour. Clients are thus enabled to assess their decisions and options, keep what is working for them, and change what is not. As a strengths-based, non-pathologizing therapeutic approach (Jones-Smith, 2013,

p. 12), NAP accentuates the strengths that the autistic individual brings to their situation often identifed by reflecting on the resilience required in their daily life, and by recognizing and valuing the common features of autism/neurodivergence. This way of working often surprises autistic clients, whose previous experiences in therapy have typically been problem-focussed and behaviourally based. They have also often been traumatic – a factor that requires the therapist's awareness and careful attention, from the initial contact. In my clinical experience, the majority of autistic adults arrive in therapy dragging an extremely heavy bag of erroneous and unhelpful beliefs about themselves, others, and the world. Generally, most of the contents of this metaphorical bag have been absorbed from other people, and some were gathered by the individual's personal experiences with navigating neuronormativity. It can take many sessions to fully unpack the bag, but it must be unpacked in service of the client's mental health, no matter how long it takes nor how circuitous the process.

Autistic strengths

Autistic individuals are just so – individuals, each with their own strengths and challenges, their own goals and obstacles, and their own story. At risk of generalizing, there are a number of truly remarkable traits and abilities that often show up in autistic individuals, which easily inform an authentic, clinically applicable, strengths-based perspective of autism.

Autistic students and employees are often highly observant, and extremely detail-oriented in their approach to work or learning. Many autistic individuals have extraordinary capacity for expansive thinking, creative ideas and unique approaches to problem-solving. In the academic world, many autistic individuals excel in fields that require logical and mathematical thinking, while many others stand out for their exceptional creativity in language, musical and artistic pursuits. In my clinical practice, most autistic clients fared significantly better than neurotypicals during the lockdown periods of the COVID pandemic because of their ability to work effectively and efficiently in relative isolation. Many autistic people are highly sensitive, and these individuals' appreciation for sensory-based experience generously enriches their own and others' lives. A strengths-based perspective of autism/neurodivergence emphasizes such valuable features as excellent semantic memory (retention and recall of details and facts), heightened pattern awareness (recognition of connections between seemingly unrelated things), and hyperfocus (capacity to focus attention deeply and for long periods). Many of the autistic people I have known (personally, as well as professionally) are resilient indiviuals who view life through a truly unique set of lenses, made from a durable blend of idealism, rationality, and fairly dark humour; their capacity to use humour to cope with experiences that would overwhelm most neurotypicals is remarkable. Additionally, autistic individuals regularly demonstrate universally valued relational behaviours including loy-alty, honesty and authenticity; often animal lovers, they are regularly described by those who know and love them as truth tellers, steadfast partners, trusted employees, and beloved, lifelong friends.

ADHD strengths

ADHD is widely recognized as a stand-alone diagnosis, and is highly prevalent among the autistic population; individuals with both diagnoses may self-identify as an "autistic extrovert", or similar. The co-occurrence of ADHD with autism is variously estimated between 30% and 80% (Leitner, 2014; Panagiotidi et al., 2019; Reiersen & Todd, 2008). Individuals with ADHD can become highly inspirational leaders who excel in motivating and encouraging other people. They are conversational experts, and often skilled negotiators and debaters. Depending on their specific type of ADHD (hyperactive/impulsive, inattentive, or combined), many ADHD-ers are known for their creativity and spontaneity; they are intensely curious and often have an insatiable drive for variety and adventure. A strengths-based perspective of ADHD values the abundant energy and unique perspectives and insights that ADHD/neurodivergent individuals bring to every situation, along with their original, outside-the-box thinking and creative problem-solving abilities.

Case conceptualization

As a backdrop to case conceptualization in NAP, clinicians and students are encouraged to explore counter-narratives to problem-saturated, neuronormative perspectives of autism/neurodivergence. A growing body of literature now exists both through intentional, autistic-led advocacy initiatives and from the wider neurodivergent community. The contributions of autistic researchers, authors and lived experts such as Layle (2024), Neff (2024), Price (2022), Nerenberg (2020), Grandin and Panek (2014) and Simone (2010a, b) supports the rationale and underscores the need for neurodiversity-affirming psychotherapy as a core clinical competency for mental health clinicians.

In psychotherapy, case conceptualization allows the therapist and client to identify a mutually acceptable definition of the problem, from where the therapist may propose a treatment plan to enable the client to make desired change. Gehart (2010, p. 17) describes case conceptualization as "the thera-peutic art of viewing … [that]enables therapists to generate new perspectives that enable them to be helpful to clients." Generating fresh perspectives of the client's situation is particularly pertinent in NAP because so many neu-rodivergent clients come to therapy with a current problem wrapped up in a complicated history that has misunderstood, disregarded or pathologized their lived experience. Sperry (2005a, b) proposes a straightforward approach to case conceptualization, outlining three central questions to be addressed by the therapist and client together: What happened? Why did it happen? How can it be changed?

NAP approaches case conceptualization from a client-focused perspective because the neurodivergent individual's experience within the dominant culture is integral to the meaningfulness of the therapist's proposed treatment plan. Along with the client's worldview, the therapist's awareness of common autistic strengths and of the impacts of neuronormativity on individuals, are prerequisates for neurodiversity-affirming case conceptualization. As Sperry (2005a, p. 358) confirmed, "The greater the similarity between [client and therapist] conceptualizations, the more likely that collaboration will occur, leading to positive treatment outcomes."

NAP and diagnosis

Neurodiversity is not a DSM-5 (American Psychiatric Association, 2022) diagnosis – it is a non-medical term that includes many brain-based diagnoses and, importantly, also includes any individual who self-identifies as such. Self-identification as neurodivergent emerges from repeatedly noticing that one's own brain processes information differently from other (neurotypical) individuals. Sensory experiences that others find pleasurable are experienced as aversive; other people's ideas of fun are dull or irritating, and (especially for autistic individuals) those same people are often unenthusiastic about one's own interests; relationships seem to have vague and inconsistent rules that cannot be broken without serious ramifications; patterns and visual details that are obvious to oneself go unnoticed by others, and so on. The experience of self-identification is a lengthy process of self-exploration and reflective practices, which may or may not be validated by a diagnosis if the individual chooses to seek assessment.

Diagnosis of mental health conditions using DSM-5 (APA, 2022), International Classification of Diseases-10 (ICD-10), or other diagnostic tools, is outside the scope of practice of most psychotherapists, apart from those who hold additional qualifications as a diagnosing physician. Nonetheless, a word about two diagnoses that fall under the umbrella of neurodiversity is pertinent: namely ASD and ADHD. Gordon Langill (2024[3]) noted that the optimal use of diagnosis is to inform treatment planning, and highlighted the importance of psychotherapists' awareness of the recommended treatments and interventions for both ASD and ADHD. This is additionally pertinent to mental health in situations where a specific treatment is mandated or requested, or when working with clients who already have a history of clinical treatment.

In settings where a specific treatment is prescribed by default, psychotherapists must think critically about the degree to which the recommended treatment for a specific diagnosis is likely to be effective for the individual client (or at least more effective than no treatment at all). As such, the psychotherapist needs assurance that the treatment is safe, and will not retraumatize the client; clarity that it is fully understood and consented to by the client or their decision-makers; and confidence that providing it is within their own clinical competencies. This is particularly pertinent when working with autistic clients, for whom a behaviourally based treatment may have been recommended by the diagnosing physician.

Regardless of the treatment plan, it is critical that non-diagnosing mental health clinicians recognize and highly value the impact of their unique role as professional listeners; educated, skilled, and compassionate hearers; and bearers of the client's story. Diagnosis may inform but does not dictate, a specific treatment plan – assuming clinical competency, this is at the discretion of the therapist. From the perspective of NAP, a diagnosis of ASD or ADHD provides one point of reference, if the client shares it with the therapist; however, it does not overshadow the client's own narrative, nor their lived experience. Clients who have had aversive clinical experiences – misdiagnosis, hospitalisation, inappropriate or ineffective medication, uninformed psychotherapy, etc. – need assurance that in the absence of danger to themselves or others; all treatment decisions (including the pace at which it progresses) will be collaborative. In sum, in psychotherapy a proposed or confirmed mental health diagnosis has a place in the clinical notes at minimum; wherever else it may be included, or excluded from therapy, remains discretionary.

Diagnostic criteria for autism

Emphasizing that diagnosis is beyond the scope of practice for most psychotherapists, this chapter highlights differing perspectives of autism, through medical and non-medical lenses. As such, an overview of the DSM-5 (American Psychiatric Association, 2022) diagnostic criteria for autism is apposite. Awareness and understanding of a client's current and previous mental health diagnoses enriches case conceptualization. A mental health diagnosis and the client's way of holding it in their own life provides important context for their experience and the meanings they attach to it. From the client's perspective, a mental health diagnosis may constitute a gift or an obstacle (or both) to their wellbeing and may carry significant weight, or very little, in their self-concept. From the therapist's perspective, it may inform (but not determine) the treatment plan and is an important element of forming a fulsome impression of the individual's life experience.

For reference purposes, the DSM-5 (APA, 2022) framework for diagnosis of autism (Autism Spectrum Disorder, ASD) requires the individual to experience persistent difficulties in the three following domains of social communication/interaction: social-emotional reciprocity, non-verbal social communication, and the ability to develop, maintain and understand relationships. They must also demonstrate at least two types of "restricted interests or repetitive behaviors" (American Psychiatric Association, 2022) from the following list: repetitive motor movements, insistence on sameness, highly restricted, fixated interests (often deemed unique or unusual), and hyper/hypo-reactivity to sensory stimuli. Diagnosticians initially identify the above criteria, and then assign a level between one and three, indicating the degree of support they assess the autistic individual requires, for optimal quality of life. Three additional factors are considerations: the symptoms must have been observable in early childhood, must cause "clinically significant impairment in social, occupational or other important areas of current functioning" (American Psychiatric Association, 2022) and the difficulties the individual is experiencing cannot be attributable to intellectual disability or global developmental delay.

Of note, individuals who meet DSM-5 criteria for a diagnosis of ASD level one (APA, 2022) would have received a diagnosis of Asperger's Syndrome from DSM-IV (in use between 1994 and 2013). Consequently, autistic adults often self-identify as having Asperger's Syndrome, rather than autism. Additionally, DSM-5 (APA, 2022) provides an additional neurodivergent diagnostic consideration: individuals who have difficulty with using language in ways that work well to establish and maintain friendships and relationships (with neurotypicals), and do not meet the other criteria for ASD, may be diagnosed with Social Communication Disorder (American Psychiatric Association, 2022).

Diagnostic criteria for ADHD

Given the prevalence of co-occurring ASD and ADHD, an overview of the diagnostic criteria for Attention Deficit Hyperactivity Disorder (ADHD) is pertinent here. Depending on the presentation of symptoms, DSM-5 (APA, 2022) diagnosis of ADHD includes three categories: hyperactive/impulsive, inattentive and the combined type, which includes features of the other two. Previously, DSM-IV referred to inattentive ADHD as Attention Deficit Disorder (ADD), which is now considered outdated terminology.

With recognition of neuronormativity and negativity within the criteria, an extensive list of potential ADHD features guides the observer and diagnostician, including the following:

Hyperactive/impulsive features:

1. Fidgets, taps, or moves a lot
2. Frequently leaves seat in meetings/classroom

3. Runs, climbs, bounces at socially inappropriate times
4. Difficulty managing leisure time or activities
5. Behaves as if "driven" or "always on the go"
6. Talks excessively
7. Blurts answers before question is complete
8. Difficulty awaiting turn
9. Interrupts or intrudes on others

Inattentive features:

1. Makes mistakes/misses details
2. Difficulty sustaining attention
3. Seems to not be listening, even when spoken to directly
4. Doesn't follow instructions/directions
5. Difficulty organizing tasks/projects
6. Avoids tasks requiring sustained effort
7. Loses necessary or important items
8. Easily distracted by extraneous stimuli
9. Forgetful of daily activities

Additionally, the symptoms of ADHD must have been observable for at least 6 months, be present in two or more settings, interfere with academic, social, or occupational functioning, and have been noted before age 12. They cannot occur exclusively during psychosis, nor be better explained by another diagnosis (e.g. Personality Disorder, Substance Intoxication or Withdrawal). And, similar to diagnosis of ASD, the diagnostician will specify whether the impacts of ADHD on the individual's daily functioning are considered mild, moderate, or severe, and treatment will be recommended accordingly.

From a mental health perspective, regardless of the specific combination of features an individual experiences, in a neuronormative culture, ADHD is often unwelcome. Along with their stated and unstated goals, individuals with ADHD carry their sensory needs, plus a long and complicated history of being in trouble for having the kind of brain they have, for errors of judgement and impulsivity in important relationships, and for underachievement in their education and career history, into the therapy room.

Neurodivergent individuals commonly request psychotherapy to address relational difficulties in their personal and professional relationships. The literature on attachment indicates that an inability to form and sustain healthy relationships is a painfully isolating experience (Hughes, 1997; Rushton et al., 2010; Zeanah & Gleason, 2015). Positive relationships are typified by back-and-forth interactions – communicative exchanges of opinions, ideas, emotions, perspectives – that meet the human needs for autonomy, competence, and relatedness

(Tang et al., 2013; Vanhee et al., 2016). However, the capacity to engage fluidly in these kinds of interactions across neurotypes is compromised by diagnostic features of ASD and ADHD, causing extensive human suffering.

Diagnosis is an individual decision. Although some parents decide against diagnostic assessment, a diagnosis of autism can provide a child with access to funding and experiences which they otherwise would not have, which is particularly pertinent to families with socio-economic obstacles to wellbeing. Such opportunities may include attending and fully participating in summer camp; receiving occupational therapy to mitigate sensory processing issues; support with school-based advocacy; participation in recreational activities with peers who share their particular interest; and, if needed, play-based, NAP, and/or parent counselling.

Additional diagnostic concerns arise because neurodivergent adults often encounter obstacles to accessing assessments for autism, causing significant frustration for adults who want to follow this path. Adult assessment is expensive, and not every community has a qualified diagnostician, so waitlists are often very long.

Diagnosis of ADHD often leads to a discussion on medication, between individuals and their doctors. Along with a blend of personalized and evidence-based strategies, many neurodivergent individuals use prescription medications for ADHD, and other co-occurring diagnoses. Psychotherapists provide a higher quality of care with a general understanding of what these medications are, how they work, and their common (or concerning) side effects. From a safety perspective, when working with clients who use medication, it is important for psychotherapists to recognize and highlight indicators that an individual should be referred to the prescribing physician for review.

Notes

1 https://neurodiversity2.blogspot.com/p/what.html
2 www.theguardian.com/world/2023/jul/05/the-mother-of-neurodiversity-how-judy-singer-changed-the-world
3 G. Langill (personal communication, February 16, 2024).

References

Ainsworth, M. D. S., Blehar, M. C., Waters, E., & Wall, S. (1978). *Patterns of attachment: A psychological study of the strange situation.* Lawrence Erlbaum.

American Psychiatric Association. (2022). Diagnostic and Statistical Manual of Mental Disorders (DSM-5-TR). In *Diagnostic and Statistical Manual of Mental Disorders.* American Psychiatric Association. https://doi.org/10.1176/APPI.BOOKS.978089 0425596

Baumeister, R., & Leary, M. (1995). The need to belong: Desire for interpersonal attachments as a fundamental human motivation. *Psychological Bulletin, 117,* 497–529.

Bottema-Beutel, K., Kapp, S. K., Lester, J. N., Sasson, N. J., & Hand, B. N. (2021). Avoiding ableist language: Suggestions for autism researchers. Autism in Adulthood, 3(1).

Bowlby, J. (1988). *A secure base: Parent-child attachment and healthy human development.* Basic Books.

Crenshaw, K. (2013). Demarginalizing the intersection of race and sex: A black feminist critique of antidiscrimination doctrine, feminist theory and antiracist politics. In K. Maschke (Ed.), *Feminist legal theories* (pp. 23–51). Routledge.

Erikson, E. (1959). *Identity and the life cycle.* International Universities Press.

Gehart, D. R. (2010). *Mastering competencies in family therapy: A practical approach to theories and clinical case documentation.* Brooks/Cole.

Grandin, T., & Panek, R. (2014). *The autistic brain: Helping different kinds of minds succeed.* Mariner Books.

Henley, A. (2013). The necessity of belonging and other discoveries. In Chang, J. (Ed.), *Creative Interventions with Children: A Transtheoretical Approach*, (pp. 12–19). Family Psychology Press.

Hughes, D. A. (1997). *Facilitating developmental attachment: The road to emotional recovery and behavioral change in foster and adopted children.* Jason Aronson.

Jones-Smith, E. (2013). *Strengths-based therapy: Connecting theory, practice and skills.* Sage Publications.

Layle, P. (2024). *But everyone feels this way: How an autism diagnosis saved my life.* Hachette Go.

Leitner, Y. (2014). The co-occurrence of autism and attention deficit hyperactivity disorder in children–what do we know? *Frontiers in Human Neuroscience, 8*(268).

Neff, M. A. (2024). *Self-care for autistic people.* Simon & Schuster.

Nerenberg, J. (2020). *Divergent mind: Thriving in a world that wasn't designed for you.* HarperOne.

Panagiotidi, M., Overton, P. G., & Stafford, T. (2019). Co-occurrence of ASD and ADHD traits in an adult population. *Journal of Attention Disorders, 23*(12), 1407–1415.

Price. D. (2022). *Unmasking autism: Discovering the new faces of neurodiversity.* Harmony.

Reiersen, A. M., & Todd, R. D. (2008). Co-occurrence of ADHD and Autism Spectrum Disorders: Phenomenology and treatment. *Expert Review of Neurotherapeutics, 8*(4), 657–669. https://doi.org/10.1586/14737175.8.4.657

Rogers, C. R. (1959). A theory of therapy, personality, and interpersonal relationships as developed in the client-centered framework. In S. Koch (Ed.), *Psychology: A study of a science* (Vol. 3). McGraw Hill.

Rushton, A., Monck, E., Leese, M., McCrone, P., & Sharac, J. (2010). Enhancing adoptive parenting: A randomized controlled trial. *Clinical Child Psychology and Psychiatry, 15*(4), 529–542.

Schmeck, K., Schlüter-Müller, S., Foelsch, P. A., & Doering, S. (2013). The role of identity in the DSM-5 classification of personality disorders. *Child and Adolescent Psychiatry and Mental Health, 7*, 1–11.

Simone, R. (2010a). *Asperger's on the job: Must-have advice for people with Asperger's or high functioning autism and their employers, educators, and advocates.* Future Horizins.

Simone, R. (2010b). *Aspergirls: Empowering females with Asperger syndrome*. Jessica Kingsley Publishers.

Sperry, L. (2005a). Case conceptualization: A strategy for incorporating individual, couple and family dynamics in the treatment process. *American Journal of Family Therapy, 33*, 353–364.

Sperry, L. (2005b). Case conceptualizations: The missing link between theory and practice. *The Family Journal, 13*(1), 71–76. https://doi.org/10.1177/1066480704270104

Strunz, R. M. (2018). Common factors of a transtheoretical model of Autism Spectrum Disorder-informed psychotherapy. *Canadian Journal of Counselling and Psychotherapy, 52*(3).

Tang, N., Bensman, L., & Hatfield, E. (2013). Culture and sexual self-disclosure in intimate relationships. *Interpersona: An International Journal on Personal Relationships, 7*(2), 227–245.

Vanhee, G., Lemmens, G., & Verhofstadt, L. L. (2016). Relationship satisfaction: High need satisfaction or low need frustration? *Social Behavior and Personality: An International Journal, 44*(6), 923–930.

Zeanah, C. H., & Gleason, M. M. (2015). Annual research review: Attachment disorders in early childhood–clinical presentation, causes, correlates, and treatment. *Journal of Child Psychology and Psychiatry, 56*(3), 207–222.

Chapter 3

Neurodiversity and the therapeutic alliance

The key to successful therapeutic outcomes is the establishment of the therapeutic alliance. This premise is additionally applicable in NAP where neurotypical therapists and neurodivergent clients seek to bridge a culturally ascribed and supported divide. In this chapter, neurotypical clinicians (particularly, but not exclusively) are invited to identify and challenge their beliefs or misconceptions about neurodivergence, Autism Spectrum Disorder (ASD), and/or attention deficit hyperactivity disorder (ADHD). Specific issues that neurodivergent individuals frequently bring to psychotherapy are highlighted, and the concept of masking as a coping mechanism among autistic individuals is illuminated. This chapter additionally informs case conceptualization and treatment planning for neurodivergent clients in psychotherapy and counselling.

Chapter 2 responds to the following clinical questions:

1. What are some of the common beliefs/misconceptions about neurodivergence that cause or exacerbate mental health challenges, in this population?
2. How do neurotypical psychotherapists intentionally deepen the *therapeutic alliance* with neurodivergent clients?
3. What does the term *masking* refer to? What is the impact of this coping mechanism on mental health in neurodivergent individuals?
4. What issues do neurodivergent clients commonly bring to therapy, that may be distinct from those that neurotypical clients bring?

In common parlance, one hears platitudes to the effect that "nobody likes change", in response to which one is moved to mention that some of us, namely psychotherapists and counsellors, make our living (and greatly enjoy doing so) by intentionally proposing, guiding, supporting, and eliciting the process of change – the same one that, purportedly, nobody likes. Perhaps it is more reasonable to propose that, "nobody likes change, *except psychotherapists*". It is fortunate indeed that therapists find change less aversive, or perhaps more intriguing, than do other people because generally, individuals come to psychotherapy seeking to make some kind of change (and requesting support to

DOI: 10.4324/9781003430476-3

navigate the process). Cozolino and Santos highlighted how the fundamental tools of psychotherapy help humans navigate the responses of our brains to life's challenges: "Due to their very complexity, our brains are extremely vulnerable to dysregulation, dissociation, and emotional distress. Fortunately for us, we possess the tools to heal one another—communication, trusting relationships, and empathy" (2014, p. 157). Effective psychotherapy involves adept and timely use of communication, trust, and empathy by a trained professional, in a safe environment, and in ways that are accessible to the specific individual who has requested help.

Psychotherapy involves verbal and non-verbal interactions that are intentionally framed to facilitate desired change (and may also facilitate unanticipated change, in and around the client!). Changes may occur in some (or all) of the cognitive, emotional, spiritual, or physical domains, and may be perceptible by others, or not. They may occur immediately or over a lengthy period, and often occur incrementally, like a snowball tumbling down a snow-covered mountain. The changes that happen in psychotherapy will affect the client, and are likely to also impact their family, friends, colleagues, and others with whom they interact, whether such individuals are consciously aware of it or not. In addition, the change that happens for the client also impacts the therapist, professionally, and even personally, because of their own engagement and active involvement with the individual and the therapeutic relationship. Corey described "a process of engagement between two people, both of whom are bound to change in the therapeutic venture." (2013, p. 7). Given the profound and widespread impact of this remarkable human endeavour, it is essential that the psychotherapist's tools – communication, trust, and empathy (Cozolino & Santos, 2014) – are consistently available, carefully honed and maintained, and judiciously used. These are the tools with which psychotherapists create and maintain enough safety for change to occur in clients and in themselves.

The specific nature or content of the change desired by clients in therapy is often a moving target, dynamically changing in emphasis and even in direction, as the process moves forward. Some clients can articulate the changes they are seeking from the start of therapy, and many cannot. Some have already tried to make the change happen themselves and encountered unexpected and seemingly insurmountable obstacles. Others feel intimidated by the perceived magnitude or complexity of the problem, feel ill-equipped or unsafe to tackle it alone, and seek help to navigate the process without becoming overwhelmed. Psychotherapists also occasionally encounter clients who are not truly seeking change but have been obliged or coerced to attend therapy by somebody else; most agree that this arrangement is unlikely to have positive outcomes; it is somewhat comparable to taking pain medication because a friend has a headache! Psychotherapy is a collaborative venture, requiring insight, commitment, and active engagement of both client and therapist to facilitate desired change.

In my experience, the kind of change that genuinely IS hard (if not impossible) for both client and therapist, is change that is not actually wanted by the client. When change occurs in psychotherapy, it happens within, and because of, the unique relationship that forms between the therapist and client. This extraordinary healing relationship is referred to as the *therapeutic alliance* (Bordin, 1979); its pivotal role in successfully facilitating desired change for the client is such that, without it, therapy devolves into a pleasant (or unpleasant) conversation, at best.

The therapeutic alliance

The therapeutic alliance, the working relationship between therapist and client, is well-established as one of the best predictors of positive outcomes in psychotherapy (Horvath & Luborsky, 1993; Martin et al., 2000). This makes sense from an attachment perspective (Bowlby, 1988); the therapeutic alliance provides a safe container for the process of change. Between client and therapist, when the alliance is robust, deep exploration is possible, risks can be taken, and myriad interactions and exchanges can occur, without damaging the integrity of their unique bond of trust and mutual respect.

Bordin (1979) articulated three components of the therapeutic alliance that facilitate the collaborative work of therapy, proposing that their very presence already constitutes an important mechanism of change. These are (a) bonds, the emotional relationship between client and therapist; (b) tasks, collaboration with therapeutic activities; and (c) goals, agreement on the expected or anticipated outcomes of therapy. Further to this, Wampold (2015) posited that at the initial meeting, new clients make extremely quick decisions about whether the therapist is trustworthy, competent and will take the time required to understand their unique story and the context in which it is set. Indeed, that initial meeting is critical; Connell et al. (2006) highlighted that more premature terminations of therapy occur after the first session than at any other point in the process. These insights are particularly pertinent for neurotypical therapists who are intending to work with neurodivergent clients; it is a privilege to hold space and time for another person's personal journey, and additionally so when therapist and client are bringing different neurotypes to the therapeutic alliance.

The therapeutic alliance between a neurotypical therapist and a neurodivergent client differs from the alliance between two neurotypical (or two neurodivergent) individuals in these same roles. Particularly when working with autistic individuals in psychotherapy, it is important for neurotypical therapists to remain curious and open to the possibility of different, and possibly unfamiliar, experiences of connection. This requires recognizing and releasing the therapist's own need for a perceptible *emotional* connection (Bordin, 1979) and to value whatever experience of connection and co-regulation is available with this client, especially in the early days. It is a common mistake for a neurotypical therapist to assume that their interpretation of an autistic client's emotional self-expression – which may feel/appear atypical or muted through a neurotypical lens – necessarily reflects the client's level of engagement with any accuracy. Equally, it is important for the neurotypical therapist to recognise that the ways in which an autistic client initiates an interaction, or maintains a back-and-forth exchange, will differ from neurotypical social communication. Openness, respect, and curiosity toward the client and for themselves underlie the appropriate therapeutic stance, optimizing the conditions for the nascent therapeutic alliance between a neurotypical therapist and a neurodivergent client. Whether or not these brain-based communication differences constitute problems for the neurodivergent client in daily life will clarify as the alliance deepens; the important point is that since establishing the therapeutic alliance is the critical task at the start of psychotherapy, the neurotypical therapist must simply appreciate the extant differences in social and emotional communication between neurotypical and neurodivergent individuals.

Returning to Bordin (1979), in Neurodiversity-Affirming Psychotherapy (NAP) it is appropriate to challenge or refute the requirement that the therapist and client form an *emotional* connection, per se. It remains critical that a connection of some nature is formed, and it remains true that it is predominantly the therapist's responsibility, at least initially, to facilitate its formation. This connection, however, may be emotional, cognitive, or spiritual in nature; it is not limited to the emotional domain. Neurodivergent clients may find it more accessible to connect with their therapists on a cognitive level initially, or even on a spiritual level, and multiple kinds of client-therapist connections are plausible soil in which to plant the seeds of the therapeutic alliance. This connection allows the therapist and client to collaboratively generate goals for the work, and enables the therapist to propose a pathway by which they might pursue those goals. Whether the bond is emotional or cognitive is less critical than whether it is safe, authentic, and sustainable. For this reason, NAP emphasises unusual elements such as the sensory environment of the therapy room, the availability of executive functioning supports and the therapist's own capacity for self-awareness and self-regulation, as accessibility requirements in cross-neurotype psychotherapy. Indeed, proposing an inaccessible pathway may arguably constitute a microaggression (Sue et al., 2007), unintentionally hurting the client, and setting the nascent therapeutic alliance on a rocky, downward spiral, from which it is unlikely to recover.

Clearly, for a robust therapeutic alliance to form between two individuals who bring different neurological arrangements, different experiences with social communication, and different sensory experience, something *different* will be required of the therapist! It is not the neurodivergent client's responsibility to adapt their self or their story to fit into a neuronormative therapeutic framework. Indeed, this experience is likely to retraumatize the client (Ecker et al., 2024) by emulating the lived experience that has contributed to their suffering and brought them to therapy in the first place. Neurodivergent advocates often articulate that their mental health problems feel like inevitable outcomes of the interminable experience of having to adapt their behaviour, suppress their needs, reduce their expectations, and compromise their aspirations to meet neuronormative societal expectations (Saunders, 2018). It is unethical to provide psychotherapy to a neurodivergent client that carries an agenda, overt or otherwise, of requiring them to behave, communicate or interact in ways that are intended to make them appear neurotypical – that is behavioural modification; it is not psychotherapy.

How can a neurotypical psychotherapist ensure everything possible has been done to ensure that the therapeutic alliance is seeded in neurodiversity-affirming ways, considering the above? One essential competency is the therapist's capacity and willingness to tolerate their own uncertainty, and to self-regulate rather than react to it. This is a difficult undertaking for most therapists because we tend to be highly motivated (not to mention trained and credentialled!) to DO something to reduce the client's suffering. NAP practice requires us to simply BE with the individual and the problem; to *resist jumping* into the deep water to save them; *to not know* what is needed; and to *intentionally self-regulate* before anything else. This capacity is foundational to the cross-neurotype therapeutic alliance, because most neurodivergent individuals carry a heavy backpack of lived experience into therapy, much of which has large elements of "fixing" (by authority figures and discriminatory systems) deep within it. NAP offers a distinctly different relational experience to the neurodivergent individual, one in which they are neither deficient nor broken, and therefore not in need of repair. Rather, this therapeutic relationship features genuine curiosity, acceptance, validation, and celebration of the neurodivergent individual's deepest self. The therapist's capacity to continuously self-regulate in response to their own uncertainty conveys non-verbally that the client is seen and accepted, that the relationship is available, and safe, and has the potential to ease their suffering by facilitating the change they desire.

According to the literature, trepidation arises for neurotypical psychotherapists in response to requests for therapy from individuals who self-identify (or are identified by the referrer) as autistic/neurodivergent. Brookman-Frazee et al. (2012) reported that psychotherapists perceive working with autistic kids as "challenging and frustrating," attributing their reluctance to work with neurodivergent kids to limitations in their own training. This highlights the tremendous need for NAP training/learning opportunities, within and beyond clinical training programs. It is incumbent on practicing mental health clinicians to self-reflect, seek clinical supervision, and hold themselves accountable, when they encounter resistance within themselves to a specific client group. This is critical within NAP because rejection is a common experience for autistic children (Jones et al., 2022). Consequently, many autistic individuals work hard to conceal their autism by adopting masking or camouflaging techniques from early childhood (Sedgewick et al., 2021), often at significant cost to their mental health. Research findings by Cage, Di Monaco, and Newell (2018) demonstrated that low levels of autism acceptance, both personally and from external sources, significantly predicted depression among neurodivergent individuals. Obviously, it is the ultimate irony when a therapist's unexamined biases, fears or assumptions become another source of rejection for an autistic/neurodivergent individual seeking psychotherapy.

A second protective factor for the therapeutic alliance between a neurotypical therapist and a neurodivergent client is the therapist's *recognition of fundamental differences* between their own mind and that of the client. The neurodiversity-affirming therapist intentionally and continuously resists assuming that the client's mind is responding similarly to their own, either around the client's own history or to their shared experience in therapy. Certainly, the therapist and client may be experiencing and interpreting their interactions similarly, but equally they may not. Again, respectful curiosity on the therapist's part is key to establishing a bi-directional flow of effective communication. This has important implications for case conceptualization; reflecting on the client's strengths and needs in such pivotal domains as sensory processing, communication and executive functioning requires the therapist to maintain a self-regulated, curious stance, cloaked in unconditional positive regard (Finlay, 2021; Rogers, 1949) for how the neurodivergent client's mind processes and responds both similarly and differently to their own. (Timulak and Keogh, 2017, p.1556) proposed that

> therapist willingness to seek client perspectives, openness to hear what clients have to say, non-defensiveness in the face of negative feedback, and ability to modulate actions accordingly are all likely to contribute to stronger relationships with clients and stronger collaboration, correspondingly contributing to stronger therapeutic outcomes.

This is as applicable in NAP as it is in every other client-centred, therapeutic framework; it may even be additionally applicable, to offset the heightened risk of premature rupture of the alliance in cross-neurotype therapeutic relationships.

Specific to psychotherapy with diagnosed individuals

Mental health clinicians are unlikely to hold the same assumptions and biases that neurodivergent individuals encounter in the wider culture, some of which will be discussed in the next section. However, there is one notable area in which counsellors and psychotherapists may be prone to neurotypical bias, shutting down their own curiosity, and compromising the client's access to therapy accordingly. This high-risk domain is in case conceptualization for clients with diagnosed neurodivergence, including ASD, ADHD, and various other DSM-5 diagnoses (American Psychiatric Association, 2022). Autistic adults regularly advocate for healthcare providers to recognise that receiving a diagnosis of autism does not, in and of itself, imply that they are sick, unhappy, needing and/or seeking treatment of any kind. Unlike many other DSM-5 (APA, 2022) diagnoses, it is distinctly possible for a mentally healthy individual to meet the diagnostic criteria for autism while living a full and joyful life, engaging in deeply loving relationships, excelling in education, parenting, career, and other meaningful life pursuits. For this reason, psychotherapists are cautioned against assuming that an autistic individual who requests therapy considers being autistic a problem – much less to be The Problem! It is entirely possible that the client's identity as a neurodivergent individual is one of their greatest sources of resilience and support. Most therapists would concur that the best way to find out what a client considers to be the problem, is to ask them; likewise, the only reliable way to find out how an autistic individual feels about being autistic, is to ask!

Conversely, within and beyond the clinical world, autistic/neurodivergent individuals frequently experience significant trauma as they navigate the school and healthcare systems, public and private alike, through childhood and adolescence. Daily, these individuals are subjected to a plethora of commonly held myths and misconceptions about who they are, what they can or cannot do, or what they do or do not need. Some of the more commonly held misconceptions and biases are articulated below, many of which would clearly have a significant negative impact on any individual's mental health during their formative years. Notwithstanding the availability of information and options for connection with others online, if not in real life, many autistic adults are relatively unaware of the extent to which such biases have impacted their own lives, reduced their opportunities to participate fully in learning opportunities, hampered their personal relationships, limited, or disrupted their careers and undermined their mental health. While anger and sadness are natural responses to this deepening self-understanding, neurodivergent individuals often report that simply identifying in psychotherapy the damaging beliefs and systemic obstacles they have encountered and navigated can facilitate a profoundly helpful shift toward self-awareness, self-acceptance, and self-compassion.

Neurodiversity: exploring the myths

Some examples of common myths around neurodiversity are provided below:

Myth: *Autism is always accompanied by atypical intelligence, either academic brilliance or intellectual disability.*

Fact: There is a range of intellectual abilities across the autistic population; Charman et al. (2011) demonstrated *limited evidence* of a distinctive IQ profile, among autistic research participants. Additionally, the results of measuring IQ in neurodivergent individuals using instruments and under test conditions that were designed for use with neurotypicals yields questionable results, in terms of validity/reliability.

Myth: *Autistic individuals neither want nor need friendships or intimate relationships.*
Fact: Autistic individuals need the support and enjoyment of meaningful friendships and relationships just as do neurotypicals. Benford and Standen (2009) demonstrated that autistic individuals are interested and motivated to connect with other people but often encounter social difficulties in effectively doing so. Additionally, Bauminger and Kasari (2000) explored loneliness and friendship in autistic children, concluding that autistic kids experience loneliness both more frequently and more intensely than their non-autistic peers.

Myth: *Autism is a diagnosed disorder that requires treatment and/or behavioural modification "cures" autism.*
Fact: Autism is a DSM-5 (American Psychiatric Association, 2022) diagnosis, which may or may not be experienced as problematic by the autistic individual. The extent to which any individual grows up in an atmosphere of unconditional positive regard and acceptance, at home, at school and in the community, serves to scaffold and strengthen their mental health. That said, the combined impacts of relational trauma, behaviour modification and adverse childhood experiences (ACEs) (Boullier & Blair, 2018) that are often associated with receiving a diagnosis of autism, plus the impacts of neuronormativity, may certainly undermine mental health. ACEs include child maltreatment, household dysfunction, community dysfunction and peer dysfunction/property victimization (Karatekin & Hill, 2019) – all of which predicate mental health difficulties in children. Additionally, the statistics around disproportionate victimization of neurodivergent kids by peers and adults demonstrate where the problems lie, and the urgency with which systemic change is needed.

Myth: *Sensory processing differences are an additional complication, rather than a central element, of neurodiversity.*
Fact: Sensory processing differences are integral aspects of neurodiversity, and thus are critical elements of case conceptualization and treatment planning in NAP.

Myth: *Selective mutism only occurs in children; selective mutism is a choice made by the neurodivergent individual to avoid engagement or demand.*
Fact: Autistic adults or children experience selective mutism, where the ability to communicate verbally is suddenly and temporarily lost in response to high

demand. Selective mutism demonstrates anxiety and should be treated as such, using trauma-informed strategies, in psychotherapy. The term "selective" is sometimes misconstrued to mean that the individual *chooses* to withdraw from verbal communication; its correct interpretation is that the sudden loss of speech occurs in a specific situation or environment. *Situational mutism* is a more accurate term that is in increasingly common use.

Myth: *Therapeutic conversations must focus on the client's particular interests or areas of expertise, and inviting the client to venture elsewhere will inevitably rupture the therapeutic alliance.*

Fact: Autistic individuals may regularly raise their particular interests in conversation, within or beyond therapy. Usually, these interests are sources of comfort, excitement, joy, or fascination for the individual, and such personal supports are welcome in the therapy room. In NAP, clients are encouraged to explore a balance of familiar and unfamiliar material, and they may choose to reference their particular interests to self-regulate in stressful or challenging moments. Autistic individuals may need additional supports such as a little extra time, or a clear request, to shift their attention elsewhere if limiting the frequency or duration of referrals to their particular interests is one of their therapeutic goals. If it is not, it is the therapist's privilege to invite the client to explore the role of their interests in promoting or undermining their mental health – and it is the client's privilege to decide what, if anything, they wish to do with the discoveries thus made.

Myth: *Somatic or vocal tics or repetitive behaviours should be suppressed or concealed by the client, either within or beyond therapy.*

Fact: Many neurodivergent individuals experience Transient Tic Disorders (TTD) and Tourette's Syndrome as co-occurring disorders. *Tics* may be obvious (sudden, visible movements or audible utterances) or less so (teeth grinding, repetitive thoughts, toe clenching, etc.). The literature on the benefits of ignoring versus suppressing tics is inconclusive; Comprehensive Behavioural Intervention for Tics (CBIT) was reported to reduce tic frequency more effectively than simply ignoring tics (Specht et al., 2013) and it was also noted that *prolonged* suppression of tics did not have the same impact. Additionally, the mental health impact of self-rejection, which is implied in tic suppression, raises concern in the context of NAP. Neurodivergent clients who identify tic suppression as a therapeutic goal may be referred to a therapist who specializes in CBIT or a comparable intervention. Those who are not pursuing this goal may wish to explore the mental health impacts of their tics while working in NAP on self-insight and self-acceptance. Clients who wish to explore medication for tics should be referred to their prescribing physician. Importantly, *Repetitive behaviours* differ from tics; a diagnostic criterion of autism, they are often described by neurodivergent clients as sources of comfort or self-regulation. Clients may find that repetitive movement (pacing, leg bouncing, fidgeting) facilitates thinking and/or self-expression, and these movements are welcomed in NAP. If clients relate that their need for movement is problematic outside of therapy, they may want to experiment with alternative movements such as doodling, sipping water, or hand/foot massage to see if similar outcomes occur; conversely, they may prefer to explore self-advocacy and consider lifestyle changes to better align their careers or living arrangements with their sensory needs.

Coping mechanisms and belonging

In response to life's challenges and adversities, people develop coping mechanisms, which (ideally) serve to buffer the effects of stress on the individual, and to enable them to move through both transient and prolonged times of difficulty. Such mechanisms include healthy pursuits such as listening to music, walking in nature, daily reflective practices and similar. They also include less-healthy behaviours such as nail biting, disordered eating, substance abuse, and self-harm. It is appropriate clinical practice for therapists and clients to reflect on the degree to which a specific coping mechanism or style may be adaptive, maladaptive, or both for an individual at a specific juncture in their lives.

Neurodiversity-affirming psychotherapists reflect on clients' coping mechanisms through a compassionate and non-judgmental lens; the same coping mechanism that is currently causing problems for a client, has usually at some point in the past been salvatory. Coping mechanisms must not be criticized; the therapist's role includes naming, validating, and investigating them with the client. Within the safety of the therapeutic alliance, it is the client's prerogative to assess whether the mechanism is currently needed and helpful to them, whether it works in the context of their present life, and at what cost to themselves or others. It is also the client's prerogative to decide whether they want to continue using a particular coping mechanism in challenging moments, to set it aside in favour of another approach, or to make adaptations to offset its costs or augment its benefits, and then continue to use it. The coping mechanism referred to as *masking*, which is commonly employed by autistic individuals to cope with their day-to-day experience, is appropriately viewed through this lens of non-judgment and unconditional acceptance.

There is little debate on the importance of connection between humans for optimal mental health; we are tribal creatures by nature (Clark et al., 2019) and to isolate us from one another is cruel indeed. Solitary confinement has long been recognized as severe punishment for incarcerated individuals, whose ability to experience belonging in society is already curtailed. The global mental health crisis that has emerged in the wake of the COVID pandemic attests to the impact of prolonged isolation on the mental health of individuals, families, and communities across the world (Ganesan et al., 2021). Additionally, a clear association has been established among loneliness, social isolation, and reduced expectations of longevity (Hajek & König, 2021). Clearly, we humans need contact with one another to be our best selves.

From a mental health perspective, it is important to note that feelings of connection with others do not necessarily arise as a direct outcome of simply being in their presence, physically or virtually. Clients who are managing loneliness or isolation, either as elements of depression or as discrete experiences, often report the painful sensation of feeling "alone in a crowd" (Comber, 2023). Humans need a *sense of belonging* to a group or of *mattering* within a community, for mental health (Adler, 1928). Lambert et al. (2013) identified that an individual's sense of belonging predicts how meaningful they perceive their life to be. This is important, because beneath so many issues that arise in therapy – grief, relational strain, work-life balance, anxiety, stress management, and physical illness – lies the need for belonging, and the quest for a meaningful life. To varying degrees, humans need one another to navigate the storms, to celebrate the joys, to experience the warmth of belonging, and thus to be assured that their own life is meaningful, while it is happening.

Alongside this need for belonging, we are an adaptive species; if we cannot meet our need for belonging simply by being who we are in a certain situation, we consciously or unconsciously avoid the pain of isolation by adapting. And, since it is easier to adapt oneself than it is to adapt a complex situation, the human brain is equipped with the capacity for neuroplasticity (Doidge, 2007). Unlike other organs in the human body, which grow and change in response to time – the brain grows and changes in response to experience. Neuroplasticity allows the brain to dynamically rewire its own neurological pathways, in both helpful and unhelpful ways, in response to our experiences (and to the meaning we assign to them) throughout our lives. We strengthen our preferred neural pathways by frequently doing things in the same or similar ways, while those we no longer need or appreciate gradually weaken and fade through lack of use. Neuroplasticity enables humans to respond to our lived experience, to learn new things, to create beauty and invent solutions – and to adjust our coping mechanisms when needed. If we are struggling with feelings of isolation or rejection in our lives, and having difficulty developing a sense of belonging, neuroplasticity enables us to adopt ways of being that we believe will result in a greater sense of acceptance by the tribe. In the neurodiversity context, this process of adopting behaviours that do not come naturally to the individual is referred to as masking; from a neuroplasticity perspective, it often becomes a significantly greater part of an individual's identity than a simple, reversible, social adaptation.

Bullying and neurodivergence

The pivotal role of peer relationships in healthy child and adolescent development is well documented, as are the devastating impacts of bullying in those same life stages. Bullies intentionally seek to harm, exclude, or intimidate their targets, and are often very subtle and calculated in how they do so. Cardinal elements of bullying include an imbalance of power (real or perceived) between bully and victim, and that the harmful behaviour is both intentional and repetitive (Menesini & Salmivalli, 2017). The negative impacts of bullying are always psychological, and are often also physical, emotional, and spiritual. As well as the painful impacts of bullying on peer relationships and mental health in childhood or adolescence, bullying in childhood is associated with the development of mental health issues in adulthood, including depression, anxiety, and suicidality (Copeland et al., 2013).

Autistic kids are bullied by peers at three to four times the rate of neurotypical kids, with negative impacts on their academic, social, and physical functioning (Hoover & Kaufman, 2018). Autistic advocates are aligned in their conviction that this happens to neurodivergent kids, literally because they are somehow different from their peers. As defined by Olweus (2013), bullying is aggressive behavior that is repetitive, intentional, and hurtful, either physically or emotionally. The sense of exclusion it engenders in the victim is a cruel antithesis of the sense of feeling involved with and integral to a system or environment (Hagerty et al., 1992) that is foundational to belonging, mental health and stability.

Devastatingly, neurodivergent children are bullied and ostracised by peers significantly more frequently than neurotypical children (Twyman et al., 2010). The dark underbelly of the need to belong is that those who are perceived by the majority as "different" become targets for bullying. Autistic kids have difficulty with reciprocal social communication, impacting peer relationships, highlighting differences between them and the neurotypical majority, and making them vulnerable to being targeted by bullies (Fink et al., 2018; Van Roekel et al., 2010). Those with co-occurring ADHD may have poor self-inhibition, increased risk-taking, and difficulties with placing and maintaining their attention on shared activities, making it difficult for them to connect in positive ways with their neurotypical peers (Twyman et al., 2010). The increasingly complicated social fabric of school, along with the highly demanding sensory environment and the ever-increasing demand on a neurodivergent student's executive functioning capacity, often makes school a highly aversive environment. Many autistic kids adapt to this environment by masking (Chapman et al., 2022), with the hope of reducing the degree of rejection they experience in the school setting. Masking can be understood as an adaptation to a child's frequent experiences of social rejection and ostracism; it is a natural response to a painful, pervasive sense of non-belonging.

Masking

Masking, the process of building an external facade to suppress or conceal one's autistic traits, is a personal process of adaptation and acculturation, intentional or otherwise. For many autistic/neurodivergent individuals, it involves some blend of camouflaging one's innate social communication style, compensating for one's executive functioning difficulties, and minimizing one's sensory needs. It may also include minimizing or concealing one's areas of particular expertise. Masking involves concealing and replacing whatever features of autism one can, by carefully watching and emulating the behaviour of neurotypical individuals.

Masking has been described as consciously or unconsciously suppressing one's natural responses and adopting alternative responses across a range of domains, which includes social interaction and sensory experience (Pearson & Rose, 2021). Price described masking as part of a "messy, unstable scaffolding of flawed coping mechanisms that autistic individuals build around themselves to hide the excessive cognitive and emotional demands placed upon them by regular life" (2022, p. 98). Masking is intended to increase the neurodivergent individual's sense of belonging, and to reduce frequent experiences of rejection, exclusion, and discrimination. The devastating impact on a child's mental health of repeated rejection by peers, and experiences of betrayal by the adults on whom they depend, often precipitates masking. Ostracism undermines a child's self-esteem and threatens their sense of belonging, personal efficacy, and meaningful existence (Pearson & Rose, 2021). It makes sense that a child who has any possibility of hiding behind a well-constructed mask to avoid such painful experience will do so, regardless of the cost to their own wellbeing.

Botha et al. (2022) highlighted the mental health impacts of masking reported by autistic adults who shared that their entire childhoods were spent trying to assimilate, or fit in, and repeatedly failing to do so. Hull et al. (2017) illustrated key elements of the process they refer to as "social camouflaging", as follows: it is motivated by the desire to fit in and to increase social connections; it comprises several techniques, which include masking and compensating; its consequences include exhaustion, challenging stereotypes, and threats to self-perception. Unsurprisingly, masking/social camouflaging have been associated with elevated stress, low mood, poor self-esteem, exhaustion, anxiety, and depressive symptoms (Hull et al., 2017) both in the moment, and cumulatively.

It is widely recognized in psychotherapy that hiding or disguising one's emotions is a natural adaptation for children who grow up in families where emotional self-expression feels unsafe or unacceptable. In attachment-based therapy with adults, much of our clinical work entails helping clients recognize the ways in which they were discouraged by primary attachment figures from feeling or expressing emotion, and working with them to reengage with, learn from, and communicate their own inner lives. For neurodivergent adults, whose emotional self-expression in childhood probably differed from that of their neurotypical peers or siblings, these feelings of discouragement or overt rejection by adults and peers were often experienced many times daily (Feldman et al., 2022). In almost every context of their lives, neurodivergent kids are literally or implicitly silenced, diminishing their sense of themselves, thwarting their development of emotional self-expression, lowering their self-esteem, and heightening self-doubt and anxiety in the process.

Abraham Maslow (1954) positioned belonging in third place in the hierarchy of human needs, preceded by physiological and safety needs. And Michael White, creator of Narrative Therapy, observed that "extremes of behaviour in children are often associated with a lack of inclusion, frequently arising in the context of severed connections with significant others" (1994, p. 51). Clearly, people need to feel a sense of belonging within the contexts of their own lives. Given their sensory processing differences in the context of the loud, fast, bright societies in which we live, it is no surprise that because of their ongoing, repeated attempts to assimilate, neurodivergent kids regularly become neurodivergent adults with extraordinary masking (social camouflaging) abilities. In fact, many of them mask so well and so long that they become unrecognizable even to themselves, and therapy consists of providing a return journey to find out just who they were, and are, beneath the weighty layers of camouflage they carry and wear each day. Holliday-Willey (2015) spotlighted the high cost of this apparent resourcefulness, highlighting that the stress that ongoing masking places on the neurodivergent individual regularly foreshadows longer-term mental health difficulties (Holliday-Willey, 2015).

Unsurprisingly, autistic kids who are good at masking grow up to be autistic adults who are good at masking, sometimes to the extent that they are masked even from themselves. With surprising frequency, parents whose kids have received a diagnosis of autism begin to wonder, and investigate, their own neurotype; autism is demonstrated to have moderate genetic heritability (Hallmayer et al., 2011); one rarely meets an autistic individual whose family tree is entirely devoid of others! Gentle investigation of early life experience is an invaluable therapeutic conversation with autistic clients who grew up in family cultures that included what I refer to as *intergenerational masking.*

Autistic children can become extremely skilled at emulating neurotypical individuals 24/7, consequently flying below the radar of parents, teachers, and medical professionals. Insidiously, masking is regularly welcomed and reinforced by neurotypical people, because it makes neurodivergent individuals "compliant and easier to deal with" (Price, 2022, p. 99). Masked individuals often remain undiagnosed and more importantly, unsupported around their sensory, communication and executive functioning needs, throughout childhood and into the adult years. This is a particularly common story for female-identifying autistic adults, as described by a client in my own practice, for example, Hailey[1]

My brother's ADHD was much *louder* than my autism. He was diagnosed and accommodated from about 5 years of age, while my needs just weren't noticed by our parents, because I was so quiet. I just cried a lot and went to my room. Everything fell apart in my first year of university. I was so used to concealing and suppressing my needs and complying with other people's demands, that I found myself living with a Stranger (who I didn't like very much) that eventually turned out to be Me.

Unmasking, or "dropping the mask" is no simple matter. Autistic individuals expend a massive amount of energy and time developing and wearing their masks, to cope with the social and sensory demands of the neurotypical world. Over time, the mask often becomes indistinguishable from their true identity and they may need extensive time and support in psychotherapy to begin to explore who they are, when masked and unmasked, and what they might want to do with these personal discoveries. From a psychotherapeutic perspective, letting down one's mask is akin to the experience of the LGBTQ2S+ individual who has long been "in the closet" and is considering "coming out", and it requires the same degree of respect, compassion, and support in psychotherapy and beyond. Autistic individuals who intend to unmask in some or all areas of their lives need ample time and support to consider the implications of doing so, and to reflect on the implications of not doing so. Likewise, those who are not yet considering "dropping the mask", even for short periods within the therapy room, must retain control over whether, why, when, and how this may happen, in their own lives. Masking and unmasking are issues of personal identity – the mask an autistic individual presents to the world was formed in response to relational trauma, and has functioned to some degree as a support for the individual in navigating the neurotypical world. Recognizing, exploring, and potentially letting it drop, either completely or partially, is complex personal work, requiring trauma-informed, neurodiversity-affirming, therapeutic support.

Common issues in NAP

The range, depth, and complexity of issues that neurodivergent clients present in psychotherapy are as varied as those presented by neurotypical clients. In my experience, neurodivergent clients who believe that their own neurological arrangement is problematic have usually grown up in families or cultural milieus that have persistently framed neurodivergence as such. For these individuals, repeated experiences of exclusion and inaccessibility in their family, school, and elsewhere have reinforced damaging messaging about neurodivergence, which was inevitably absorbed by the individual. From childhood, neurodivergent individuals are scapegoated for marital, family, school, and even societal problems. The truth is that discriminatory policies emerging from inaccurate, outdated information result in problem-saturated narratives within the healthcare and educational systems. Unless they are masked to the extent that they are silent and invisible, neurodivergent children and youth are seen as inherently challenging, and treated accordingly, with devastating outcomes.

As mentioned previously, neurodivergent clients request psychotherapy for similar reasons that neurotypical clients do – anxiety, depression, overwhelm, expired or ineffective coping mechanisms and so forth. However, there are some specific issues that arise almost uniquely for neurodivergent clients. In general, these difficulties arise from the lived experience of neurodivergent individuals in a predominantly neurotypical culture. Examples of commonly arising problems include:

(a) deciding whether to seek assessment for adult diagnosis of ADHD or ASD, and considering the potential impacts of "late diagnosis" on oneself and others
(b) choosing whether/when to manage one's ADHD with lifestyle strategies, medication, or a blend of both
(c) exploring/accepting one's sensory profile; recognizing its impact on mental health to date; investigating it's impacts on self-regulation
(d) recognizing one's own intersectionality: neurotype; gender; sexuality; Black, Indigenous, and People of Colour (BIPOC); socio-economic status; etc.
(e) expressing grief/anger around previous misdiagnoses (often with serious psychiatric disorders); understanding impacts of associated therapies and treatments (hospitalization, medications etc.)
(f) examining the mental health impact of executive functioning difficulties such as time management, organization style and distractibility
(g) making neurodiversity-affirming decisions around life tasks such as partnering, education, career planning, becoming a parent, etc.
(h) exploring masking, camouflaging, identity, and advocacy issues
(i) Identifying/addressing self-regulatory issues: sleep disorders, gastrointestinal disorders (irritable bowel syndrome [IBS]), disordered eating, food allergies or sensitivities, etc.
(j) exploring emotional experience/difficulties: anxiety, perfectionism, depression, loneliness, anger, perceived inadequacy, shame, etc.

An array of specific strategies that will be helpful to neurotypical therapists in unpacking and exploring such issues with clients in neurodiversity-affirming ways, is offered in Chapter 9. However, in concluding this chapter, it is essential to reemphasize the centrality of the therapist's stance and demeanour, over and above any specific strategy or intervention, in providing psychotherapy that is accessible and helpful to neurodivergent clients. The contextual model of psychotherapy proposed by Imel and Wampold (2008) beautifully depicted psychotherapy as a particular kind of "social healing practice", highlighting the pivotal role of establishing the therapeutic alliance as the foundation for the subsequent social communication exchanges through which the client's healing is facilitated. In NAP, as in all attachment-based therapies with the neurotypical therapist's commitment to establishing and sustaining the therapeutic alliance in neurodiversity-affirming ways, it is perfectly reasonable to anticipate seeing the proverbial "Dodo Bird" (Rosenzweig, 1936) peacefully waddling into view over the horizon, in the fullness of time.

Note

1 Not her real name.

References

Adler, A. (1928). *Die Technik der Individual-Psychologie*. Bergmann.

American Psychiatric Association. (2022). *Diagnostic and statistical manual of mental disorders*. American Psychiatric Association. https://doi.org/10.1176/APPI. BOOKS.9780890425596

Bauminger, N., & Kasari, C. (2000). Loneliness and friendship in high-functioning children with autism. *Child Development, 71*(2), 447–456. https://doi.org/10.1111/1467-8624.00156

Benford P., & Standen P. J. (2009). The Internet: A comfortable communication medium for autistic people? *Journal of Assistive Technologies, 3*(2), 44–53.

Bordin, E. S. (1979). The generalizability of the psychoanalytic concept of the working alliance. *Psychotherapy: Theory, Research & Practice, 16*(3), 252–260..

Botha, M., Dibb, B., & Frost, D. M. (2022). "Autism is me": An investigation of how autistic individuals make sense of autism and stigma. *Disability and Society, 37*(3), 427–453. https://doi.org/10.1080/09687599.2020.1822782

Boullier, M., & Blair, M. (2018). Adverse childhood experiences. *Paediatrics and Child Health, 28*(3), 132–137. https://doi.org/10.1016/J.PAED.2017.12.008

Bowlby, J. (1988). *A secure base: Parent-child attachment and healthy human development*. Basic Books.

Brookman-Frazee, L., Drahota, A., Stadnick, N., & Palinkas, L. A. (2012). Therapist perspectives on community mental health services for children with autism spectrum disorders. *Administration and Policy in Mental Health, 39*(5), 365. https://doi.org/10.1007/S10488-011-0355-Y

Cage, E., Di Monaco, J., & Newell, V. (2018). Experiences of autism acceptance and mental health in autistic adults. *Journal of Autism and Developmental Disorders, 48*, 473–484.

Chapman, L., Rose, K., Hull, L., & Mandy, W. (2022). "I want to fit in... but I don't want to change myself fundamentally": A qualitative exploration of the relationship between masking and mental health for autistic teenagers. *Research in Autism Spectrum Disorders, 99*, 102069.

Charman, T., Pickles, A., Simonoff, E., Chandler, S., Loucas, T., & Baird, G. (2011). IQ in children with autism spectrum disorders: Data from the Special Needs and Autism Project (SNAP). *Psychological Medicine, 41*(3), 619–627. https://doi.org/10.1017/S0033291710000991

Clark, C. J., Liu, B. S., Winegard, B. M., & Ditto, P. H. (2019). Tribalism is human nature. *Current Directions in Psychological Science, 28*(6), 587–592. https://doi.org/10.1177/0963721419862289

Comber, C. (2023). *The intersection of loneliness and counselling from a pluralistic perspective, using a hermeneutic approach* [Doctoral Dissertation]. ResearchSpace@ Auckland.

Connell, J., Grant, S., & Mullin, T. (2006). Client initiated termination of therapy at NHS primary care counselling services. *Counselling and Psychotherapy Research, 6*(1), 60–67.

Copeland, W. E., Wolke, D., Angold, A., & Costello, E. J. (2013). Adult psychiatric outcomes of bullying and being bullied by peers in childhood and adolescence. *JAMA Psychiatry, 70*(4), 419–426. https://doi.org/10.1001/JAMAPSYCHIATRY.2013.504

Corey, G. (2013). *Theory and practice of counseling and psychotherapy* (9th ed.). Cengage Learning/Brooks Cole.

Cozolino, L. J., & Santos, E. N. (2014). Why we need therapy-and why it works: A neuroscientific perspective. *Smith College Studies in Social Work, 84*(2–3), 157–177. https://doi.org/10.1080/00377317.2014.923630

Doidge, N. (2007). *The brain that changes itself: Stories of personal triumph from the frontiers of brain science*. Penguin.

Ecker, B., Ticic, R., & Hulley, L. (2024). The transformational psychotherapy of emotional unlearning. In B. Ecker, R. Ticic, and L. Hulley (Eds.), *Unlocking the emotional brain* (pp. 44–78). Routledge.

Feldman, M., Hamsho, N., Blacher, J., Carter, A. S., & Eisenhower, A. (2022). Predicting peer acceptance and peer rejection for autistic children. *Psychology in the Schools, 59*(11), 2159–2182. https://doi.org/10.1002/PITS.22739

Fink, E., Olthof, T., Goossens, F., van der Meijden, S., & Begeer, S. (2018). Bullying-related behaviour in adolescents with autism: Links with autism severity and emotional and behavioural problems. *Autism, 22*(6), 684–692. https://doi.org/10.1177/1362361316686760

Finlay, L. (2021). *The therapeutic use of self in counselling and psychotherapy*. Sage Publications.

Ganesan, B., Al-Jumaily, A., Fong, K. N., Prasad, P., Meena, S. K., & Tong, R. K. Y. (2021). Impact of coronavirus disease 2019 (COVID-19) outbreak quarantine, isolation, and lockdown policies on mental health and suicide. *Frontiers in Psychiatry, 12*. www.frontiersin.org/journals/psychiatry/articles/10.3389/fpsyt.2021.565190/full#h4

Hagerty, B. M. K., Lynch-Sauer, J., Patusky, K. L., Bouwsema, M., & Collier, P. (1992). Sense of belonging: A vital mental health concept. *Archives of Psychiatric Nursing, 6*(3), 172–177.

Hajek, A., & König, H. H. (2021). Do lonely and socially isolated individuals think they die earlier? The link between loneliness, social isolation and expectations of longevity based on a nationally representative sample. *Psychogeriatrics: The Official Journal of the Japanese Psychogeriatric Society, 21*(4), 571–576. https://doi.org/10.1111/PSYG.12707

Hallmayer, J., Cleveland, S., Torres, A., Phillips, J., Cohen, B., Torigoe, T., Miller, J., Fedele, A., Collins, J., Smith, K., Lotspeich, L., Croen, L. A., Ozonoff, S., Lajonchere, C., Grether, J. K., Risch, N., Cleveland, M., & Cohen, M. (2011). Genetic heritability and shared environmental factors among twin pairs with Autism HHS public access. *Archives of General Psychiatry, 68*(11), 1095–1102. https://doi.org/10.1001/archge npsychiatry.2011.76

Holliday-Willey, L. (2015). *Pretending to be normal: Living with Asperger's Syndrome (Autism Spectrum Disorder)*. Jessica Kingsley.

Hoover, D. W., & Kaufman, J. (2018). Adverse childhood experiences in children with autism spectrum disorder. *Current Opinion in Psychiatry, 31*(2), 128–132.

Horvath, A. O., & Luborsky, L. (1993). The role of the therapeutic alliance in psychotherapy. *Journal of Consulting and Clinical Psychology, 61*(4), 561–573.

Hull, L., Petrides, K. V., Allison, C., Smith, P., Baron-Cohen, S., Lai, M. C., & Mandy, W. (2017). "Putting on my best normal": Social camouflaging in adults with autism spectrum conditions. *Journal of Autism and Developmental Disorders, 47*(8), 2519–2534. https://doi.org/10.1007/S10803-017-3166-5/TABLES/2

Imel, Z. E., & Wampold, B. E. (2008). The importance of treatment and the science of common factors in psychotherapy. In S. D. Brown & R. W. Lent (Eds.), *Handbook of counseling psychology* (4th ed., pp. 249–266). John Wiley & Sons.

Jones, S. C., Gordon, C. S., Akram, M., Murphy, N., & Sharkie, F. (2022). Inclusion, exclusion and isolation of autistic people: Community attitudes and autistic people's experiences. *Journal of Autism and Developmental Disorders, 52*(3), 1131–1142. https://doi.org/10.1007/S10803-021-04998-7/METRICS

Karatekin, C., & Hill, M. (2019). Expanding the original definition of Adverse Childhood Experiences (ACEs). *Journal of Child & Adolescent Trauma, 12*(3), 289. https://doi.org/10.1007/S40653-018-0237-5

Lambert, N. M., Stillman, T. F., Hicks, J. A., Kamble, S., Baumeister, R. F., & Fincham, F. D. (2013). To belong is to matter. *Personality and Social Psychology Bulletin, 39*(11), 1418–1427. https://doi.org/10.1177/0146167213499186

Martin, D. J., Garske, J. P., & Davis, M. K. (2000). Relation of the therapeutic alliance with outcome and other variables: A meta-analytic review. *Journal of Consulting and Clinical Psychology, 68*(3), 438–450..

Maslow, A. H. (1954). *Motivation and personality*. Harper and Row.

Menesini, E., & Salmivalli, C. (2017). Bullying in schools: The state of knowledge and effective interventions. *Psychology, Health & Medicine, 22*, 240–253. https://doi.org/10.1080/13548506.2017.1279740

Olweus, D. (2013). School bullying: Development and some important challenges. *Annual Review of Clinical Psychology, 9*, 751–780. https://doi.org/10.1146/ANNU REV-CLINPSY-050212-185516

Pearson, A., & Rose, K. (2021). A conceptual analysis of autistic masking: Understanding the narrative of stigma and the illusion of choice. *Autism in Adulthood, 3*(1), 52–60. https://doi.org/10.1089/AUT.2020.0043

Price. D. (2022). *Unmasking autism: Discovering the new faces of neurodiversity*. Harmony.

Rogers, C. R. (1949). The attitude and orientation of the counselor in client-centered therapy. *Journal of Consulting Psychology, 13*(2), 82–94.

Rosenzweig, S. (1936). Some implicit common factors in diverse methods of psychotherapy. *American Journal of Orthopsychiatry, 6*(3), 412–415. https://doi.org/10.1111/J.1939-0025.1936.TB05248.X

Saunders, P. (2018). Neurodivergent rhetorics: Examining competing discourses of autism advocacy in the public sphere. *Journal of Literary & Cultural Disability Studies, Liverpool University Press, 12*(1), 1–17.

Sedgewick, F., Hull, L., & Ellis, H. (2021). *Autism and masking: How and why people do it, and the impact it can have.* Jessica Kingsley Publishers.

Specht, M. W., Woods, D. W., Nicotra, C. M., Kelly, L. M., Ricketts, E. J., Conelea, C. A., Grados, M. A., Ostrander, R. S., & Walkup, J. T. (2013). Effects of tic suppression: Ability to suppress, rebound, negative reinforcement, and habituation to the premonitory urge. *Behaviour Research and Therapy, 51*(1), 24–30. https://doi.org/10.1016/J.BRAT.2012.09.009

Sue, D. W., Capodilupo, C. M., Torino, G. C., Bucceri, J. M., Holder, A. M. B., Nadal, K. L., & Esquilin, M. (2007). Racial microaggressions in everyday life: Implications for clinical practice. *American Psychologist, 62*(4), 271–286.

Timulak, L., & Keogh, D. (2017). The client's perspective on (experiences of) psychotherapy: A practice friendly review. *Journal of Clinical Psychology, 73*(11), 1556–1567. https://doi.org/10.1002/JCLP.22532

Twyman, K. A., Saylor, C. F., Saia, D., MacIas, M. M., Taylor, L. A., & Spratt, E. (2010). Bullying and ostracism experiences in children with special health care needs. *Journal of Developmental and Behavioral Pediatrics, 31*(1), 1–8. https://doi.org/10.1097/DBP.0B013E3181C828C8

Van Roekel, E., Scholte, R. H. J., & Didden, R. (2010). Bullying among adolescents with autism spectrum disorders: Prevalence and perception. *Journal of Autism and Developmental Disorders, 40*(1), 63. https://doi.org/10.1007/S10803-009-0832-2

Wampold, B. E. (2015). How important are the common factors in psychotherapy? An update. *World Psychiatry, 14*(3), 270. https://doi.org/10.1002/WPS.20238

White, M. (1994). Ritual of inclusion: An approach to extreme uncontrolled behaviour in children and young adolescents. *Journal of Child and Youth Care, 9*, 51–51.

Self- and co-regulation in Neurodiversity-Affirming Psychotherapy (NAP)

This chapter presents clinician self-awareness and intentional self-care as integral elements of Neurodiversity-Affirming Psychotherapy (NAP). It is appropriate to situate self-regulation and co-regulation at the heart of attachment-based therapies, and to emphasize the importance of these processes in neurodiversity-affirming, trauma-informed, clinical practice. The additional strain on psychotherapists who work in predominantly neuronormative settings is broached, and significant risk for compassion fatigue/clinician burnout when providing cross-neurotype psychotherapy in isolation is discussed. The interdependent processes of clinician self-awareness and self-regulation are explored, with particular focus on intentional self-care as a clinical competency within NAP.

Chapter 4 responds to the following clinical questions:

1. How does the self of the therapist impact client outcomes in NAP?
2. What is meant by *autistic mental health*?
3. What is *co-regulation*?
4. In what ways are *self-regulation* and *co-regulation* interdependent?
5. How are *vicarious trauma*, *clinician burnout*, and *self-care* managed in NAP?

Autistic mental health

Robust mental health is a desirable, valuable, and enriching element of human life. Expanding the observation that good mental health consists of significantly more than the absence of mental illness, the World Health Organization (2004) proposed the following general definition: "a state of mental well-being that enables people to cope with the stresses of life, realize their abilities, learn well and work well, and contribute to their community". This definition becomes more meaningful with explicit recognition of mental health as a culturally specific concept, requiring culturally responsive care (Snodgrass et al., 2017). Possible

DOI: 10.4324/9781003430476-4

indicators of declining mental health are appropriately assessed with a fulsome awareness of the client's social and cultural context (e.g. among recent immigrants, unemployment may indicate a language barrier rather than a decline in mental health; among neurodivergent individuals repetitive movements may indicate sensory self-care rather than a decline in mental health). Post-modern therapeutic approaches recognize that mental health is determined and impacted by a complex interplay of individual, social and structural stresses, inequalities, and vulnerabilities (World Health Organization, 2022b).

In this book, as in my clinical practice, the term "autistic mental health" refers to the pathway or process by which an autistic/neurodivergent individual is likely to reach, or return to, mental health. This pathway often differs from how a neurotypical individual would travel toward a similar destination and may also have a different starting point. This book illuminates some common differences between neurodivergent and neurotypical pathways to mental health, with the goal of normalizing them all in clinical practice. Additionally, the phrase "autistic mental health" is intended to raise awareness, to highlight the potential impacts of neuronormative assumptions in cross-neurotype psychotherapy. These impacts are mitigated by the neurotypical psychotherapist's self-awareness and accountability, while centering the neurodivergent client's personal narratives around their mental health in case conceptualization, treatment planning, and throughout the therapeutic journey. Practice-based evidence, lived experience, and the extant literature inform my current clinical position that a mentally healthy autistic individual values their own neurotype equally with all others, and lives accordingly.

Mental health exists on a continuum between optimal states of wellbeing to debilitating states of great suffering (Patel et al., 2018), and there are no one-size-fits-all descriptors for mental health, neither autistic nor allistic. Ideally, clinical diagnoses of mental health disorders situate the client's personal narrative within pertinent cultural factors, and integrates the physician's experience and observations with input from people who have known the individual across time. However, autistic advocates and clinicians have pointed out that when viewed through the lens of neuronormativity, many neurodivergent traits and behaviours (e.g. hyperfocus, echolalia, selective mutism, sensory sensitivities, reduced eye contact, self-soothing with repetitive movement, etc.) are frequently misinterpreted by diagnosticians, with serious consequences for the autistic/neurodivergent client/patient and those who love them (Au-Yeung et al., 2019; Baudino, 2010).

Pervasive neuronormativity and ableism in mental healthcare has resulted in misdiagnoses of autistic adults when diagnosticians have incorrectly attributed the individual's neurodivergent traits to serious mental health diagnoses. It has been my privilege to work with several neurodivergent individuals who have navigated the impacts and implications of weighty (and incorrect) DSM-5 (American Psychiatric Association, 2022) diagnoses including bipolar disorder, as well as borderline, schizoaffective, and antisocial personality disorders. These clients' lived experience includes hospitalization for psychiatric care, multiple trials of psychotropic medications with associated side effects, and the inevitable social/emotional ramifications of receiving a serious, often stigmatizing, mental health diagnosis. As a non-diagnosing clinician with an unwavering commitment to public safety and some insight into neurodivergence, I listen very carefully when such experiences are shared in therapy. As psychotherapists, we do not diagnose, nor do we prescribe medication. Our clinical tool is the therapeutic alliance, allowing us to centre the client's narrative about who they are, what has happened to them, and what they think might be helpful now. What matters most in attachment-based psychotherapy is that we provide the client with a safe, well-informed, co-regulated, relational experience, and that together we lean in, and explore whatever happens next.

Often catching our attention more insistently when it is depleted, than when it is robust, various indicators can suggest a decline in mental health, subjectively or objectively. Individuals of all neurotypes may report combinations of disrupted sleep, increased or decreased appetite, reduced pleasure in things they usually enjoy, episodes of anxiety or excessive worrying, prolonged self-isolation, cognitive distortions and so forth. Self-injurious behaviour and suicidal ideation are experienced by all neurotypes, although both are disproportionately prevalent in the neurodivergent population (Cassidy et al., 2014; Croen et al., 2015; Segers & Rawana, 2014).

My practice-based experience aligns with the evidence in the literature demonstrating that neurodivergent individuals are more vulnerable to fragile mental health than neurotypicals. Moseley et al. (2019) propose that alexithymia, depression, anxiety, and sensory processing issues may increase the occurrence of non-suicidal self-injury (NSSI) among autistic individuals. Cassidy et al. (2018; 2020) demonstrated that a diagnosis of autism is an independent risk factor for suicide, which they propose is exacerbated among the neurodivergent population by masking, and unmet support needs. Oliphant et al. (2020) confirmed that 66% of autistic adults have experienced suicidal ideation, and 35% have planned or attempted suicide. Kerns and Kendall (2012) highlight anxiety as one of the most commonly occurring mental health conditions in autistic individuals. Russell et al. (2013) noted the common co-occurrence of Obsessive Compulsive Disorder (OCD) and autism. It is blatantly clear that the understanding and treatment of mental health in autistic individuals, and among the neurodivergent population in general, requires the attention of researchers, commitment of clinical training programs, and clinical competency of mental health clinicians.

Asking for help

Individuals who request psychotherapy are people who have detected a decline in their own mental health, identified their need for support, and decided to request it. Often, they have already attempted to address the problem independently;

they may have had help or advice (solicited or otherwise) from friends and family but remain unsatisfied with the outcome. For many people, requesting help from a psychotherapist requires significant courage because it requires telling a stranger that one is struggling to cope with a personal challenge. And autism can considerably magnify both the degree of difficulty experienced and the degree of courage required in this moment. Requesting help is a distinct departure from the innate tendencies of most autistic individuals, whose default approach to a problem is usually to tackle and solve it, autonomously (and often with excellence!).

At the same time, gathering the courage to step beyond one's comfort zone by requesting help is a fine starting point for the therapeutic journey. The energy generated in the shift from the Contemplation to the Action stages of change (Prochaska & DiClemente, 1982) kindles a bright flame of responsiveness in most psychotherapists. Therapist responsiveness refers to the capacity and willingness of a therapist to adapt their preferred interventions or strategies to meet their clients' specific mental health needs (Wu & Levitt, 2022). Responsiveness among therapists is elegantly described by Hatcher as "a counterweight to the wish to pin things down, to be certain about what to do…" and is recognized for its importance in keeping therapists, "alert to changing conditions, new threats and opportunities, and limits to what we know and can do" (2021, p. 37). Since asking for help is less comfortable for neurodivergent individuals than for neurotypicals (who may also find it difficult) therapist responsiveness in this situation requires the therapist to ensure they are equipped to facilitate an autistic client in telling their story. There are many ways to do this, depending upon the therapist's preferred therapeutic approach(es).

Clients who have less ease with verbal self-expression or difficulty with isolating individual areas of strength and challenge may more easily describe the situation using externalizing techniques such as Sandtray/Sandplay (if they don't find the texture of sand aversive), painting, drawing or collage, or even letter writing, any of which may be excellent alternatives to a back-and-forth verbal exchange. When a conversation is available, neurodivergent clients may benefit from additional structure, such as the therapist offering some potential areas of focus. For example, the core domains of mental health articulated by Fusar-Poli et al. (2020) may help an autistic client to categorize their experience, enriching an intake conversation accordingly: (i) mental health literacy; (ii) attitude toward mental disorders; (iii) self-perceptions and values; (iv) cognitive skills; (v) academic/occupational performance; (vi) emotions; (vii) behaviours; (viii) self-management strategies; (ix) social skills; (x) family and significant relationships; (xi) physical health; (xii) sexual health; (xiii) meaning of life; and (xiv) quality of life. Not infrequently, neurodivergent individuals within my practice have reflected that their understanding of their mental health prior to entering therapy tended to be "all or nothing", including neither incremental degrees of wellness, nor identification of distinct domains. Autistic minds often have great affinity for categorizing, so framing the discussion in this way may scaffold the reflective process, allowing the individual to recognize areas where their mental health is stable or robust, as well as areas where they believe that support is needed.

Trauma and dysregulation

Much has been written about the nature of trauma, its impacts on the brain and on quality of life, and on how to recognize and care for it in psychotherapy. Trauma has been effectively described as "the lasting emotional response that often results from living through a distressing event".[1] While it varies widely among individuals, this prolonged and recurring emotional response may include a reduced sense of safety in one's life, a distorted sense of self, reduced self-awareness, and self-regulatory capacity and increased or atypical difficulty with navigating relationships. Additionally, one of the cardinal signs of a trauma response is that it often manifests as dysregulation in the individual in response to an incident or experience that others perceive as an insignificant or a non-event. For this reason, trauma responses are often minimized, even by those closest to the individual, resulting in additional suffering caused by lack of empathy and support, isolation, perceived abandonment and unsurprisingly, increased anxiety. (Purkey et al., 2018) summarized the five principles of trauma-informed clinical practice as follows: (i) bearing witness to the client's experience of trauma (also referred to as "awareness and acknowledgement"); (ii) safety and trustworthiness; (iii) choice, control and collaboration; (iv) believing in (and building on) the client's strength and resilience; and (v) sensitivity to the client's culture, ethnicity and personal and social identity. There are multiple iterations of the principles of trauma-informed care in the literature, but the summary above draws the therapist's attention to the critical elements: deep listening, relational safety, collaboration within the therapeutic alliance, recognition of resilience, and centring the client's identity within the professional caring relationship.

Self-awareness and self-regulation in the therapist

Psychotherapists create and hold space for clients to do their personal work, and their own presence and way of being in the therapeutic space is a critical common factor for change. Therapist self-awareness refers to the therapist's ability to monitor the internal state of their self, moment-to-moment, even as they are also monitoring the impact their internal state may be having on the client. Yalom (2002, p. 40) asserted that the therapist's own psychotherapy is "by far the most important part of psychotherapy training," highlighting the need for therapists to appreciate the centrality of their own self-awareness and presence within the working alliance. Fife et al. (2014) proposed that the therapist's self, their own way of being, is the foundational common factor in effective psychotherapy, upon which the alliance and the use of techniques are dependent. Baldwin (2013, p. xvi) describes the self of the therapist as "the funnel through which theories and techniques become manifest." A therapist's authentic commitment to noticing and attending to their own inner state is a prerequisite for effectively supporting a client to notice, investigate, and take care of theirs.

Closely related to self-awareness is the concept of self-regulation, which refers to intentionally doing something to attend to one's inner state, to reach or maintain a sense of inner balance. A self-aware therapist discerns and assesses slight shifts in their own internal world and takes action to up-regulate (energize themselves) or down-regulate (settle themselves), to ensure they are fully available, dynamically attuned, and appropriately responsive to the client. Unless self-regulation is the specific topic of discussion, within session the therapist's self-regulatory activity is usually unobtrusive; it might include sipping water or tea, shifting one's body position, or using a small fidget item to provide subtle tactile stimulus. Importantly however, a therapist's ability to self-regulate dynamically is dependent on multiple factors, most of which occur outside that session; effective psychotherapists improve the quality of their own presence in therapy by engaging in clinical supervision, reflective practice, professional learning, peer consultation and regular, personalized, self-care practices.

Astute self-awareness and capacity for intentional self-regulation in the therapist are additionally important to the therapeutic alliance when therapist and client have, or may have, different neurotypes. Many neurodivergent individuals are highly sensitive to dysregulation in other people, and the opportunity such individuals will have to make desired personal change through psychotherapy, will be thwarted by dysregulation in the therapist. Hypersensitivity often renders the pace and intensity of neurotypical social life exhausting for autistic individuals, making sensory processing a focal point of NAP. Such individuals regularly identify as "empaths", meaning they are acutely aware of the internal states of people around them, and often have difficulty distinguishing their own inner state from others'. Neff (2024, p. 10) described this experience: "When you're Autistic [sic], it's as if your nervous system exists on the outside of your body, fully absorbing every single sensory input, social interaction and piece of information … your internal battery is always being used, and so it depletes faster than those of your neurotypical peers". This heightened awareness of other people's emotional states and its draw on the individual's own resources has been reported or endorsed by most of the autistic clients within my practice. This highlights the necessity for therapists who are providing NAP to consistently attend to their own inner state, before and during therapy with a neurodivergent client. Happily, self-awareness and self-regulation are interdependent processes, and the ease with which a therapist recognizes their own shift towards dysregulation and effectively self-regulates improves incrementally, with regular practice and accumulated experience.

Co-regulation in psychotherapy

Co-regulation is what happens when living creatures attune to one another, and is at the root of empathy and responsiveness in relationships. Fogel (1993, p. 6) noted that co-regulation occurs when "people's joint actions blend to create a unique and mutually created set of social actions". Co-regulation is a continuous process involving two individuals whose actions are dynamically impacting one another. Gutstein (2009, p. 114) highlighted that in healthy relationships, co-regulation often occurs with either one or both partners unaware that it is happening. In the context of attachment-based psychotherapy, co-regulation between therapist and client is the glue that strengthens the therapeutic alliance, and without which the therapeutic process is unlikely to move forward.

The experience of co-regulation in therapy has some commonality with co-regulation in secure attachment relationships between parents and babies. It may be described as the process by which one (regulated) person supports another (dysregulated) person to shift to a regulated state, with both individuals positively affected by the process. Co-regulation usually occurs with minimal discussion of what is happening. Parent-infant co-regulation occurs when the baby's cry momentarily dysregulates the (regulated) parent, who responds by taking action to soothe the baby, resulting in both individuals returning to a regulated state. Co-regulation requires "attunement" Malloch & Trevarthen (2009, p. 8); parents often reflect on how the challenging early days of parenting gradually become easier, as they and their baby attune to one another through shared, mutually enjoyable interactions. In secure attachment relationships, babies communicate to parents when they are dysregulated, and parents endeavour to provide what they need – sometimes engaging in behaviours that were not previously in their repertoire: pacing, rocking, singing, and so forth. Through the rhythmic "musicality" of their connection (Malloch & Trevarthen, 2009, p. 8) the parent-baby dyad learns to co-regulate, trust is deepened, and secure attachment is established.

In many ways, the process of co-regulation between client and therapist mirrors this dynamic, from the moment the therapist becomes aware of a regulatory shift within themselves, in response to something happening in the space between them and the client. The client may be observably distressed, or not at all, but the therapist self-regulates, and wordlessly, the client is invited to attune to their inner state. And, in moments when the client is openly dysregulated, the therapist resists becoming entwined by continuing to draw on their own self-awareness and to gently self-regulate, conveying empathy and availability all the while.

This is a fine dance, often requiring every ounce of the therapist's available resources to extend a metaphorical hand from a place of inner equilibrium, through a door that is just the right size for this individual client to step through, even when dysregulation blocks their view of what is on the other side. The strength of the therapeutic alliance is tested at such moments, and the therapist's ability to continue to convey safety, unconditional acceptance and quiet encouragement to the dysregulated client, is key to its survival. As the client finds a sense of safety and inner balance, the therapist reaffirms their own inner equilibrium. Co-regulation in psychotherapy has relatively little to do with neuro-type, and everything to do with our individual presence, our shared experience and our common humanity; it is central to effective, attachment-based therapy between a neurotypical therapist and a neurodivergent client.

Co-regulation across neurotypes

Attachment theory underscores the importance of the self-regulation/co-regulation feedback loop between the therapist and client described above. It is not uncommon to hear new psychotherapists in clinical supervision confounded by a neurodivergent client's apparent difficulty with learning to self-regulate, even when the client is aware that regular or intense dysregulation has disrupted or damaged previous relationships. It is helpful to view such situations through an attachment-oriented lens, recognizing that individuals who did not have regular, easeful opportunities to co-regulate with adults in infancy, may need additional support to learn how to self-regulate later in life.

An important point requires highlighting here, because this is often the moment when a very large elephant attempts to enter the room! Bruno Bettelheim's (1967) erroneous hypothesis of autism as an outcome of relational trauma in childhood had widespread, negative impacts. Bettelheim was a survivor of the Nazi concentration camps, and this hypothesis revealed the distortion of his diagnostic lens by his own childhood trauma.[2] Consequently, even today, strident resistance arises in response to any discussion that includes autism and attachment in the same sentence, making it an unnecessarily difficult, and arguably a neglected, field of study. Should it arise for the psychotherapist, the appropriate, neurodiversity-informed response to the question is: autism is not an outcome of early life relational trauma. Autism is the expression of a neurodivergent individual's neurological arrangement (Amaral et al., 2011; Liu, 2019; Masataka, 2017; Price, 2022). Simultaneously, it is also true that cross-neurotype relationships are complex and often challenging, and when they occur between a parent and child, co-regulation is often a more complicated process than the neurotypical parent had anticipated.

Returning then, to the question of co-regulation in psychotherapy, and how best to support an individual in therapy who did not fully learn to self-regulate in childhood. If the client is autistic, and believes their parents were allistic, a small insight may be available. In relationships where one individual is neurotypical and the other neurodivergent, relational difficulties often emerge, and increasingly so if there is a power imbalance and a host of relational expectations, such as those between parents and infants. A neurotypical parent with a neurodivergent baby will likely experience some relational difficulties in the early months, requiring a particular kind of support to co-regulate with their baby. A neurotypical employer and neurodivergent employee may encounter some communication issues between them, until clarity is established. Likewise, a neurotypical therapist with a neurodivergent client requires a particular kind of self-awareness, an extensive capacity for self-regulation, and a willingness to coregulate with a client whose inner and outer experience differs significantly from their own.

While this highlights the need for therapist self-regulation prior to co-regulating with a client, it also reflects a developmental feedback loop; not only does self-regulation in one facilitate co-regulation between two, but co-regulation between two is a necessary precursor to self-regulation in one! Babies who are reliably soothed by attuned caregivers in times of discomfort, fear, or loneliness form the neurological pathways that will eventually allow them to self-soothe in healthy, adaptive ways (Sylvester & Scherer, 2022). And people who can self-soothe with relative ease, tend to have more capacity to soothe and support other people. Conversely, babies whose adults are not attuned to their needs when distressed have difficulty learning to self-sooth, and may develop different neurological pathways, showing up later in distrust of relationships, or a tendency to resist or disrupt experiences of care and connection (Hughes et al., 2019, p. 46). In attachment theory, patterns of disruptive relational behaviours are interpreted as indicators of insecure attachment; this may or may not be the case in cross-neurotype attachment relationships.

Co-regulation is an important key to reflecting on cross-neurotype psychotherapy, just as when parent and baby have different neurotypes, establishing and maintaining co-regulation may be more challenging. The core features of neurodivergence – sensory processing, communication, and executive functioning – often complicate co-regulation for neurodivergent infants with neurotypical parents. Such parents may later share that they had difficulty soothing their infant, or that they felt as if they and the baby were slightly out of sync. Hypothetically, if the neurodivergent baby could share their experience, they might report that despite their best efforts to communicate what they needed, that the parent didn't seem to be really paying attention, or similar! Assuming there is love, and the parent is adequately supported, this parent and child will develop their own version of secure attachment, sometimes with significantly more effort and frustration than occurs between parents and babies of the same neurotype. While managing the discomfort of their sensory sensitivities, the neurodivergent baby may begin to experience themself as challenging or hard to soothe, reflecting their parents' experience of feeling inadequate, frustrated or constantly exhausted. Everybody is doing their best, but the rhythm of co-regulation is very hard to find, and when found, is hard to sustain.

In this way, the beloved autistic child of allistic parents often experiences a greater degree of relational stress than a neurotypical child would experience, caused by the dynamics of the relationship itself. Secure attachment requires safety and reciprocity in the parent-child relationship (Bowlby, 1979; Crowell & Waters, 1994), both of which depend upon the parent and baby first establishing a "functional, reciprocal communication system" (Gutstein, 2009). Finding the rhythm of their unique communication system is perhaps little complicated; the music is playing, but the dancing partners keep stepping on one another's toes! It is hard, but not impossible. Emphatically, in healthy, loving, cross-neurotype, parent-infant relationships, this is not a question of love. What is also true, however, is that in my clinical experience, the themes of being loved but not understood, or of being loved but not completely seen/understood/accepted are still the most common that arise, for autistic/neurodivergent adults in cross-neurotype psychotherapy.

School-based trauma

There remains another elephant in the room, and this one really does require – nay, demand – our attention. Chapter 3 suggested some commonly arising issues that autistic clients bring to psychotherapy. With reference to the World Health Organization (2004) criteria for mental health ("cope with the stresses of life, realize their abilities, learn well and work well, and contribute to their community"), many autistic/neurodivergent clients recall rare (if any) accessible, neurodiversity-affirming opportunities to acquire the skills and experience during their school years that would have enabled them to meet any of these criteria in adulthood.

Rather, a majority of autistic/neurodivergent adults recall their school years as confusing and chaotic, and many can share clear accounts of school-based trauma, inflicted by peers, teachers, and administrators. Some recall the names of one or two memorable teachers in whose classes they were "allowed" to work within their own learning style and meet their own sensory needs; many years of consulting on neurodiversity in schools has confirmed for me that those specific teachers were either themselves neurodivergent or were either of neurodivergent kids.

With some exceptions, neurodivergent kids are regularly excluded throughout their formative years from the very experiences and activities that youth need to allow them to develop communicative resilience and social confidence; recognize and value their unique strengths and abilities; and make valued contributions to their school community. More often, neurodivergent adults in therapy recall their school years as punctuated with daily experiences of exclusion, isolation or overt bullying, communication breakdowns and misunderstandings, and sensory overwhelm. They regularly describe ways in which their own learning opportunities were limited by discriminatory policies and inadequate supports at school. For lack of understanding, resources, and appropriately qualified professionals, suspensions, expulsions, and other punitive measures are daily occurrences in schools, causing untold damage to neurodivergent students' mental health, with long-term ramifications. As expressed by one autistic client, close to the end of their Grade 12 year: "I survived high school and I'm about to graduate ... but if those were the best years of my life, I dread to imagine what will happen at university".

Therapist attachment

A chapter on attachment-based psychotherapy across neurotypes is incomplete without some reference to the impact of the therapist's own attachment style on the therapeutic alliance. It is well-established that in often unanticipated and complex ways, the quality of the alliance and the outcomes of therapy are influenced by the therapist's own attachment history (Bucci et al., 2016; Degnan et al., 2016). While several studies have supported the hypothesis that securely attached therapists have additional capacity to avoid or effectively navigate therapeutic ruptures (Mallinckrodt, 2000; Schauenburg et al., 2010), there is evidence suggesting that therapists and clients with oppositional attachment styles may also develop strong alliances (Bucci et al., 2016). The important points are ethical practice, self-awareness and professional responsibility. Therapists who develop awareness of their own attachment style are better equipped to effectively manage the inevitable activation of their attachment history within the therapeutic alliance (Rizou & Giannouli, 2020), thus protecting the alliance from premature rupture and increasing the client's opportunity for successful therapeutic outcomes.

Vicarious trauma, compassion fatigue, and burnout

The multiple causes and outcomes of burnout and compassion fatigue in psychotherapy are well-researched and equally well-documented, and the tragic outcomes of both can include disappointment, disenchantment and even departure from the profession. Vicarious trauma occurs with repeated or prolonged exposure to traumatic narratives, in the absence of adequate ways to offset this exposure. It also occurs when the therapist's ability to attune to the client's emotional or psychological state "goes awry" (Kostouros, 2017), and the therapist is injured by the experience, along with the client. In the context of attachment-based therapy, this may occur if co-regulation is not established, and repeated communication or relational breakdown occurs between client and therapist; another compelling argument for therapist selfcare in cross-neurotype psychotherapy.

Saakvitne and Pearlman (1996) asserted that it is impossible to work with survivors of trauma and not be fundamentally changed by the experience. As a result of pervasive neuronormativity in the social contexts of their lives, most neurodivergent individuals seeking psychotherapy are trauma survivors – whether the trauma is relational, physical, or emotional. The opportunity to work with trauma survivors whose neurotype differs from one's own is as rewarding as it is demanding when the psychotherapist takes responsibility for their own selfcare. However, in the absence of self-awareness and self-care, the cross-neurotype working alliance is hard work for both client and therapist, and the outcome unlikely to be positive. Along with the avoidable harm that a negative experience in therapy does to the client, such experiences also have negative effects on therapists, which eventually cumulate in compassion fatigue and clinician burnout, if ignored. The signs and symptoms of compassion fatigue among clinicians include increased negativity, reduced frustration tolerance, self-destructive behaviours, loss of hope, and detachment from family or friends. Burnout manifests as symptoms of anxiety, nightmares, difficulty separating work from personal life, and, unsurprisingly, a diminished sense of purpose in one's work, and decreased feelings of accomplishment (Kostouros, 2017). Self-awareness is a critical and effective protective factor against compassion fatigue among psychotherapists, but only when it is accompanied by the courage to care for oneself at least as well as one would care for a client who presents with similar signs and symptoms.

Given the additional complexity inherent in a cross-neurotype working alliance, the neurotypical therapist is called upon to consistently prioritize self-awareness, self-regulation and selfcare. By so doing, the therapist can provide the neurodivergent client with a co-regulated relational experience within which to pursue their therapeutic goals, without compromising their own mental health and wellbeing in the process. This is the essence of attachment-based, trauma-informed, psychotherapy between a client and therapist with different neurotypes.

Notes

1   www.camh.ca/
2   https://blogs.uoregon.edu/autismhistoryproject/people/312-2/

References

Amaral, D., Geschwind, D., & Dawson, G. (Eds.). (2011). *Autism spectrum disorders*. Oxford University Press.

American Psychiatric Association. (2022). *Diagnostic and statistical manual of mental disorders*. American Psychiatric Association. https://doi.org/10.1176/APPI. BOOKS.9780890425596

Au-Yeung, S. K., Bradley, L., Robertson, A. E., Shaw, R., Baron-Cohen, S., & Cassidy, S. (2019). Experience of mental health diagnosis and perceived misdiagnosis in autistic, possibly autistic and non-autistic adults. *Autism*, *23*(6), 1508–1518.

Baldwin, M. (2013). *The use of self in therapy*. Routledge. www.routledge.com/The-Use-of-Self-in-Therapy/Baldwin/p/book/9780415896030

Baudino, L. M. (2010). Autism spectrum disorder: A case of misdiagnosis. *American Journal of Dance Therapy*, *32*(2), 113–129.

Bettelheim, B. (1967). *The empty fortress: Infantile autism and the birth of the self*. Free Press of Glencoe.

Bowlby, J. (1979). The Bowlby-Ainsworth attachment theory. *Behavioral and Brain Sciences*, *2*(4), 637–638.

Bucci, S., Seymour-Hyde, A., Harris, A., & Berry, K. (2016). Client and therapist attachment styles and working alliance. *Clinical Psychology & Psychotherapy*, *23*(2), 155–165.

Cassidy, S., Bradley, P., Robinson, J., Allison, C., McHugh, M., & Baron-Cohen, S. (2014). Suicidal ideation and suicide plans or attempts in adults with Asperger's syndrome attending a specialist diagnostic clinic: A clinical cohort study. *The Lancet Psychiatry*, *1*(2), 142–147.

Cassidy, S., Bradley, L., Shaw, R., & Baron-Cohen, S. (2018). Risk markers for suicidality in autistic adults. *Molecular Autism*, *9*, 1–14.

Cassidy, S. A., Gould, K., Townsend, E., Pelton, M., Robertson, A. E., & Rodgers, J. (2020). Is camouflaging autistic traits associated with suicidal thoughts and behaviours? Expanding the interpersonal psychological theory of suicide in an undergraduate student sample. *Journal of Autism and Developmental Disorders*, *50*, 3638–3648.

Croen, L. A., Zerbo, O., Qian, Y., Massolo, M. L., Rich, S., Sidney, S., & Kripke, C. (2015). The health status of adults on the autism spectrum. *Autism*, *19*(7), 814–823.

Crowell, J. A., & Waters, E. (1994). Bowlby's theory grown up: The role of attachment in adult love relationships. *Psychological Inquiry*, *5*(1), 31–34. https://doi.org/10.1207/S15327965PLI0501_4

Degnan, A., Seymour-Hyde, A., Harris, A., & Berry, K. (2016). The role of therapist attachment in alliance and outcome: A systematic literature review. *Clinical Psychology & Psychotherapy*, *23*(1), 47–65.

Fife, S. T., Whiting, J. B., Bradford, K., & Davis, S. (2014). The therapeutic pyramid: A common factors synthesis of techniques, alliance, and way of being. *Journal of Marital and Family Therapy*, *40*(1), 20–33.

Fogel, A. (1993). *Developing through relationships*. University of Chicago Press.

Fusar-Poli, P., de Pablo, G. S., De Micheli, A., Nieman, D. H., Correll, C. U., Kessing, L. V., Pfennig, A., Bechdolf, A., Borgwardt, S., Arango, C., & van Amelsvoort, T. (2020). What is good mental health? A scoping review. *European Neuropsychopharmacology*, *31*, 33–46.

Gutstein, S. (2009). *The RDI book*. The Connections Center.

Hatcher, R. L. (2021). Responsiveness, the relationship, and the working alliance in psychotherapy. In J. C. Watson & H. Wiseman (Eds.), *The responsive psychotherapist: Attuning to clients in the moment* (pp. 37–58). American Psychological Association.

Hughes, D. A., Golding, K. S., & Hudson, J. (2019). *Healing relational trauma with attachment-focused interventions: Dyadic developmental psychotherapy with children and families*. WW Norton & Company.

Kerns, C. M., & Kendall, P. C. (2012). The presentation and classification of anxiety in autism spectrum disorder. *Clinical Psychology: Science and Practice, 19*(4), 323.

Kostouros, P. (2017). Shifting the effects of vicarious trauma and compassion fatigue [Public presentation], Mount Royal University.

Liu, S. (2019). Autism spectrum disorder. *Integration, 804*, 754–0000.

Mallinckrodt, B. (2000). Attachment, social competencies, social support, and interpersonal process in psychotherapy. *Psychotherapy Research, 10*(3), 239–266.

Malloch, S., & Trevarthen, C. (2009). *Communicative musicality*. Oxford University Press.

Masataka, N. (2017). Implications of the idea of neurodiversity for understanding the origins of developmental disorders. *Physics of Life Reviews, 20*, 85–108.

Moseley, R. L., Gregory, N. J., Smith, P., Allison, C., & Baron-Cohen, S. J. M. A. (2019). A 'choice', an 'addiction', a way 'out of the lost': Exploring self-injury in autistic people without intellectual disability. *Molecular Autism, 10*, 1–23.

Neff, M. A. (2024). *Self-care for autistic people*. Simon & Schuster.

Oliphant, R. Y., Smith, E. M., & Grahame, V. (2020). What is the prevalence of self-harming and suicidal behaviour in under 18s with ASD, with or without an intellectual disability? *Journal of Autism and Developmental Disorders, 50*(10), 3510–3524.

Patel, V., Saxena, S., Lund, C., Thornicroft, G., Baingana, F., Bolton, P., Chisholm, D., Collins, P. Y., Cooper, J. L., Eaton, J., & Herrman, H. (2018). The Lancet Commission on global mental health and sustainable development. *The Lancet, 392*(10157), 1553–1598.

Price. D. (2022). *Unmasking autism: Discovering the new faces of neurodiversity*. Harmony.

Prochaska, J. O. & Diclemente, C. C. (1986). Toward a comprehensive model of change. In W. R. Miller & N. Heather (eds.), *Treating Addictive Behaviors. Applied Clinical Psychology*, (vol 13). Springer. https://doi.org/10.1007/978-1-4613-2191-0_1

Purkey, E., Patel, R., & Phillips, S. P. (2018). Trauma-informed care: Better care for everyone. *Canadian Family Physician, 64*(3), 170–172.

Rizou, E., & Giannouli, V. (2020). An exploration of the experience of trainee integrative psychotherapists on therapeutic alliance in the light of their attachment style. *Health Psychology Research, 8*(3), 153–166.

Russell, A. J., Jassi, A., Fullana, M. A., Mack, H., Johnston, K., Heyman, I., Murphy, D. G., & Mataix-Cols, D. (2013). Cognitive behavior therapy for comorbid obsessive-compulsive disorder in high-functioning autism spectrum disorders: A randomized controlled trial. *Depression and Anxiety, 30*(8), 697–708.

Saakvitne, K. W., & Pearlman, L. A. (1996). *Transforming the pain: A workbook on vicarious traumatization*. WW Norton & Co.

Schauenburg, H., Buchheim, A., Beckh, K., Nolte, T., Brenk-Franz, K., Leichsenring, F., Strack, M., & Dinger, U. (2010). The influence of psychodynamically oriented therapists' attachment representations on outcome and alliance in inpatient psycho-therapy. *Psychotherapy Research, 20*(2), 193–202.

Segers, M., & Rawana, J. (2014). What do we know about suicidality in autism spectrum disorders? A systematic review. *Autism Research, 7*(4), 507–521.

Snodgrass, J. G., Lacy, M. G., & Upadhyay, C. (2017). Developing culturally sensi-tive affect scales for global mental health research and practice: Emotional balance, not named syndromes, in Indian Adivasi subjective well-being. *Social Science & Medicine, 187*, 174–183.

Sylvester, E., & Scherer, K. (2022). *Relationship-based treatment of children and their parents: An integrative guide to neurobiology, attachment, regulation, and discipline (IPNB)*. WW Norton and Company.

World Health Organization. (2004). *Promoting mental health: Concepts, emerging evi-dence, practice: Summary report*. World Health Organization.

World Health Organization. (2022b). *World mental health report: Transforming mental health for all*.

Wu, M. B., & Levitt, H. M. (2022). How to become a responsive therapist: A study of experiences of developing therapists. *Psychotherapy Research, 32*(6), 763–777.

Yalom, I. D. (2002). *The gift of therapy: An open letter to a new generation of therapists and their patients*. HarperCollins.

Chapter 5

Sensory processing and mental health

The sounds, smells, sights, tastes, and sensations that arise in our day-to-day lives are subjectively experienced, ranging from pleasant to aversive and including everything in between.

For many autistic/neurodivergent individuals, the sensory environment represents a significant territory of concern … aversive experience of the physical and social world is often intense, and for some is a significant factor affecting quality of life. In this chapter, impacts of the sensory processing features of neurodivergence on mental health are examined. Clinicians are provided with a basic understanding of sensory processing, and the ways in which sensory processing is inextricably intertwined with autistic mental health is highlighted. The importance of centring the neurodivergent client's sensory experience within the therapeutic alliance is emphasized, and clinicians are guided in how to integrate this into case conceptualization and treatment planning and delivery. This material frames awareness of sensory processing as an accessibility concern, encouraging the clinician to enact their social justice role by supporting neurodivergent clients to self-advocate around their sensory processing needs in therapy and beyond.

This chapter responds to the following clinical questions:

1. What does *sensory processing* refer to, and why is it central to autistic mental health?
2. What is *Sensory Processing Disorder*, and how does it overlap with neurodiversity?
3. How does the clinician adapt the therapeutic environment to provide Neurodiversity-Affirming Psychotherapy (NAP)?

Introducing sensory processing

We humans (of all neurological arrangements) are equipped with five senses (sight, hearing, touch, taste, smell) and three sensory systems (vestibular,

DOI: 10.4324/9781003430476-5

proprioceptive and interoceptive) (Parham & Crickmore, 2022; Shanker, 2010). Spanning a wide spectrum from pleasurable to aversive, and at varying degrees of intensity, we experience the world through a moment-to-moment flow of sights, sounds, smells, tactile sensations, and tastes; each sense expresses itself both independently and in concert with others.

Our sensory experience is unique to each of us, and it changes throughout our lives as our sense organs develop and change in sensitivity, our brain changes in interpretation, and the world around and within us presents an ever-changing array of circumstances. Young children are often entertained by exploring and comparing their sensory experiences; one may love to suck on lemons or inhale the smell of pickles, while another will find these aversive, and prefer the sweeter tastes of candy or blueberry pie. Sensory experience cannot be wrong, meaning that neither child's experience is correct nor incorrect! Their different experiences simply reflect the different ways their brains interpret and respond to the information their sense organs have conveyed – sensory experience emerges from an *ongoing process of interpretation* by the individual within whom it is occurring (Greenberg, 2004). This is why people have different preferences for sitting on hard or soft surfaces, sleeping under light or heavy blankets, inhaling the smell of a campfire, or savouring the taste of blue cheese, fresh peaches, or buttery toast. It is also the reason why individuals have varying degrees of attraction or aversion to bungee jumping, eating broccoli, cutting their nails and hair, swimming in cold water, and so forth. As the adage sagely reminds us, it would be a boring world indeed, if we were all the same!

Sensory processing informs and enriches (or disrupts) our moment-to-moment experience and is as integral to our mental health as breathing, eating, or sleeping. Throughout the day, information is constantly flowing to our brains, gathered from outside by our sense organs: ears, eyes, nose, tongue, and skin. The outer layer of the brain is referred to as the *cortex* and is divided into several function-specific areas. The *tactile sense* (touch) uses nerve endings in the skin to gather information, which is conducted and processed in the *somatosensory cortex* of the brain. Taste and smell rely on the mouth and nose to collect and transmit information for interpretation to the *olfactory and gustatory cortices*, respectively. When a dog barks, our ears collect the sound and convey it to the *auditory cortex* of the brain, where it is interpreted as the voice of a dog. When a flower blooms in our yard, our eyes collect the information and convey it to the *visual cortex*, where it is processed, compared with prior experience, and duly assigned meaning – it's a flower! Multiple other mental processes such as language (for naming the object) and memory (for associating this flower with previous ones) are involved, but for our purposes, suffice to recognize that we see the flower with our eyes, and *assess and evaluate* it with the visual cortex of our brain. Thus, our sense organs/systems and our brains are in constant conversation with one another. As we interact with the world, an endless flow of sensory information is processed and interpreted in the brain, to which we are responding or reacting with thoughts, emotions, and actions.

In addition to these five familiar senses we have three sensory systems, namely the vestibular, proprioceptive and interoceptive, which employ various individual organs and cortices to gather, interpret and respond to incoming information. The *vestibular system* relies on the eyes, ears, and tactile sense to gather information about our balance, and help us correct it when necessary. The *proprioceptive system* gathers information from muscles and joints to tell us how coordinated our movements are, how much pressure we should apply to a physical task, and where our bodies are positioned (sitting, standing, upside-down on the monkey bars, etc.) And the *interoceptive system* carries messages from within our own bodies to the brain, allowing us to feel hunger, fatigue, or sickness and to respond by taking care of ourselves accordingly. The proprioceptive, interoceptive and vestibular systems are each composed of multiple sense organs working together to keep us balanced, upright and aware of ourselves, our needs, and our safety (Parham & Crickmore, 2022).

While we might compare sensory processing to the flow of a river that cannot be dammed, it can also be likened to an unrelenting social media feed that absorbs a significant proportion of our attentional and energetic resources, every day. Indeed, we continue to receive and respond to sensory input even while asleep, making us vulnerable to disturbance or awakening in response to temperature changes, compelling sounds, or unexpected smells. It is important, therefore, to understand what is happening, how it affects us and how to engage with our own and our clients' sensory processing as a pathway to mental health and wellbeing.

In the best of times, our senses connect us with ourselves, other living creatures, and the world around us – in a steady stream of sensory experience eliciting satisfying, easeful responses. Our morning beverage, with its gently swirling colours, tantalizing aroma, warmth in our hands, and particular blend of taste, temperature, and texture … such are the pleasurable moments our senses and brain provide. Mindfulness practitioners have enriched their own and others' lives by intentionally bringing awareness to their sensory experience, and rarely do such individuals regret their chosen path. For neurodiversity-affirming therapists however, it is essential to remain curious about the individual nature of sensory experience, and to hold awareness that what is pleasurable to one person, will be less so (and may even be highly aversive) to another. Most neurodivergent individuals experience sensory hyper/hyposensitivity; recognizing this aspect of their experience, and challenging negative narratives around it, provides a critical pathway to self-acceptance and self-care. The extraordinary gifts and contributions of well-supported highly sensitive people (HSPs), some of whom are autistic and all of whom belong under the neurodiversity umbrella, has been beautifully highlighted by authors such as Elaine Aron (2013) and Susan Cain (2013).

Sensory processing disorder

Recognizing the pioneering work of American psychologist and occupational therapist A. Jean Ayres in the early 1970's, we refer to the ways that sensory information arrives and is processed, and how we respond/react to it, as *sensory integration* (or *sensory processing* (Kilroy et al., 2019). Ayres defined sensory integration as: "the neurological process that organises sensation from one's own body and from the environment and makes it possible to use the body effectively within the environment" (1972, p. 11). Clinical applications of sensory integration theory are abundant in the world of occupational therapy (OT), emerging from Ayres' original model of Sensory Integration Therapy (SIT). Initially designed for working with children, SIT is now considered a mainstream OT intervention for people of all ages with sensory processing challenges, whether from birth or because of traumatic injury to the brain or sense organs (Randell et al., 2022). These interventions aim to strengthen the connections among sensory processing and emotional regulation and behaviour (including communication), thus enhancing learning, enriching experience, and enabling personally meaningful participation in daily life. Taking a brain-based, somatic (body-centred) approach to optimising wellbeing and improving physical function enables occupational therapists to reduce discomfort, alleviate anxiety, remediate symptoms of Post-Traumatic Stress Disorder (PTSD) and Complex PTSD, and enhance the client's capacity to effectively regulate their emotional and physiological arousal levels (Machingura & Lloyd, 2017; Sutton et al., 2013). From a psychotherapeutic perspective, it is easy to understand how awareness and improvements in the quality of sensory processing are likely to positively impact mental health, presenting a compelling argument for collaborative practice between occupational therapists and psychotherapists when supporting autistic/neurodivergent clients.

Most neurodivergent individuals navigate daily life with one or more sensory processing challenges (Morgan, 2019), which is referred to as Sensory Processing Disorder (SPD) or Sensory Integration Disorder (SID), in clinical settings. Since these processing differences do not appear in the DSM-5 (American Psychiatric Association, 2022) as discrete diagnoses, they are often overlooked by the medical community, although "hyper or hyporeactivity to sensory input" is a noted diagnostic feature of autism. One common example of SPD in neurodivergent individuals is *misophonia*, which manifests as strong emotional responses (often anger or anxiety) to certain sounds, often those of other people chewing, swallowing, or breathing (Kumar et al., 2017). The social and familial impacts of misophonia are significant, and support may be minimal if awareness of the brain-based nature of this sensory processing disorder is lacking, in individuals or their families.

Many neurodivergent individuals have reduced *interoceptive awareness* which manifests as muted awareness of their own internal sensations of hunger, fatigue, a full bladder or rectum, muscle tension, and so on. This brain-based difficulty with noticing and interpreting one's physiological state or needs (which is a common precursor to dysregulation) reduces the probability of neurodivergent individuals recognizing their need to take breaks from focussed or high-demand activities. Taking intentional breaks (from work, school, parenting, and other life tasks) to rest the brain and meet one's need for food, movement, rest, hydration, and other physiological imperatives, is a non-negotiable mental health requirement for autistic/neurodivergent individuals. Many clients effectively use routine, to ensure their own self-care in this area.

Autistic author Jenara Nerenberg (2020) wrote powerfully about the self-insight she has developed from understanding and meeting her own sensory needs, sharing that "feeling at home for me [sic] means being able to sink into a space beyond my own body, a kind of oneness with a room, a place or even a person" (2020, p. 148). Within my own clinical practice, I have yet to meet a neurodivergent individual who does not experience some (usually a significant) degree of stress, fatigue, or overwhelm related to sensory processing. Most neurodivergent clients experience significant relief when we validate this issue, explore it together in therapy, and reposition it at the core of their personal mental health selfcare, to be carried forward after therapy is concluded.

Sensory dysregulation and psychotherapy

Recognizing the centrality of sensory processing to mental health for neurodivergent individuals, it is critical that we effectively integrate this awareness into case conceptualization and treatment planning for neurodivergent clients. In individual ways, we humans are innately oriented toward achieving and maintaining a sense of inner equilibrium; we don't thrive on imbalance (Phillips, 2010). In periods of our lives when we feel unbalanced, physically, or psychologically, reestablishing a sense of balance quickly becomes a safety-related imperative, which few people can ignore without undesirable outcomes. Traumatised clients commonly experience feelings of physical and psychological discomfort, dizziness, fogginess, or nausea, or even difficulty breathing, when working with traumatic memories. In such moments, therapists provide trauma-informed interventions and support (Grassmann et al., 2023; Porges & Dana, 2018), intentionally creating safety and restoring a felt sense of balance, within the client. These interventions constitute psychological first aid; when a client is overwhelmed, all else must wait while we provide refuge, and as much support, space, and time as the client needs, to join us there (Levine et al., 2018).

Not infrequently, a neurodivergent client will arrive for therapy somewhat dysregulated – perhaps due to the sensory impacts of a difficult commute, a challenging day at work, or a gradual drain of their sensory resources without opportunities to decompress and self-regulate. This generally occurs more frequently in the early phases of psychotherapy before sensory self-care has been highlighted, addressed, and prioritized. The autistic client may be so accustomed to this dysregulated feeling that, for them, it is not particularly noteworthy. The attuned psychotherapist will observe that the client has difficulty settling and focussing their attention, perhaps even finding it challenging to enter the space or respond to the therapist's greeting. Conversely, they may begin speaking very rapidly, barely taking a breath between sentences, and the therapist will have difficulty interjecting! In the early days, therapists are well-advised to self-regulate, stay present, and observe these communication patterns; there will be ample opportunity to investigate them together once the therapeutic alliance is established. It is worth mentioning also that each clinician must decide for themselves how much of the content of a dysregulated individual's narrative need be documented; in the absence of safety-related information about themselves or others, I generally document sparsely during such periods, recognizing that the neurodivergent client is verbalizing to self-regulate and settle into therapy, rather than to communicate clinically important details.

In a different scenario, the client may arrive regulated but become dysregulated during the session, in response to elements of the physical environment, the therapeutic process, or their own inner world, any of which can cause or exacerbate sensory overload. Dysregulation manifests in multiple ways, some more apparent than others. Dysregulated autistic individuals may have increased difficulty with verbal self-expression and reach for a cushion or soft toy to hold or squeeze, a set of noise-cancelling headphones to wear temporarily, or a pillow to prevent additional visual input. They may cry, tremble, or become increasingly louder, may hold or compress parts of their body (clutching stomach, folding arms), or may detach or dissociate (staring, withdrawing, becoming silent, etc.) (Levine, 2016). It is important that psychotherapists recognize that asking an autistic individual to describe or explain what is happening when they are dysregulated is unhelpful, both for the client and for the therapeutic alliance. With recognition that communication is impacted in neurodivergence, doing so places an untenable additional demand on most autistic individuals, and is likely to intensify the degree of overwhelm they are experiencing. For some individuals, *selective (situational) mutism* results in sudden and almost complete inability to speak, sometimes for a prolonged period. Uninformed attempts by clinicians to force an autistic client to override this stress response will be additionally traumatising to the individual, and will not facilitate their verbal communication.

While it may be unfamiliar, the opportunity to support a significantly dysregulated autistic client is an important moment for the therapeutic alliance and is rarely an emergency. After assessing that physical safety is established, the therapist's priority is to intentionally self-regulate; we cannot help a dysregulated individual if we ourselves are not fully present and mindfully available. We might (silently) exhale a prolonged breath, bring awareness to our own grounded self, or internally re-establish the connection between our feet and the floor. Inwardly, we can remind ourselves that the client's suffering is real, and that it is temporary. In psychotherapy, this moment of self-regulation serves three main purposes; to ensure we are positioned and equipped to help; to convey recognition and acceptance of the client's distress; and to model appropriate selfcare. The therapist's calm recognition and acceptance of the client's distressing experience of sensory dysregulation is essential to their capacity to accept it themselves, later in the therapeutic journey. Often, neurodivergent children are neither taught nor permitted to attend to their own sensory needs, giving rise to many of the mental health challenges they bring into therapy as adults.

When a client becomes dysregulated in session, we may recognize an inner disruption within ourselves, a felt sense of uncertainty or discomfort, which provides information that is critical to the therapeutic alliance. Minimal clinical insight is required to recognize that some kind of relational or communication breakdown is happening, and to infer that a pause, or change of pace, is indicated. Trauma-informed psychotherapists will recognize that the client's limbic system is activated (Jackson-Perry et al., 2020) and that the freeze response has made them unable to speak, and sometimes also to move. Executive functioning – which comprises higher order cognitive processes such as thinking, organising, deciding, and planning – is inaccessible to the client at such a moment (Levine et al., 2018; Nesin-Perna, 2023); Chapter 7 explores this topic in detail.

When this happens, the therapist self-regulates and creates space, time, and physical supports for safety and comfort, while the client navigates their limbic response until their cognitive resources are available once again. What is needed is uncomplicated; we self-regulate, and then we do something intentional to help the client return to a sense of safety and balance. We may provide a weighted blanket or eye-mask and dim the lights; we might gesture toward a beanbag or swinging chair; we might offer a quiet word of reassurance while passing the client a cushion or stuffed toy to hug. Some autistic clients (not all) find guided, mindfulness-based techniques such as slow, intentional breathing or body scanning helpful. Some therapists will name the shared experience aloud, and some will simply hold space and time to sit together in quiet recognition and acceptance of what is happening. As previously stated, in NAP the therapist supports the client by self-regulating, thus creating safety. By providing safe space and ample time for self-care we model, invite, facilitate, and encourage the client to take care of themselves in accessible, sensory-based ways.

Sensory dysregulation may be obvious, or very subtle. An autistic client's ability and inclination to communicate the extent of their distress, and their associated needs, will vary. It will also vary from one instance to another within the same individual, which is a common relational issue for neurodivergent individuals who are partnered with neurotypicals. Many neurodivergent individuals have learned to internalise their emotional self-expression by masking, largely in response to adverse childhood experiences (ACEs) associated with expressing them outwardly (Barrett, 2020), at home or at school.

In contrast to many neurotypical clients, inviting a neurodivergent client to immediately reflect verbally on an experience of dysregulation is not helpful. In many cases, it is more appropriate to offer a sofa and blanket for the client to briefly nap, if possible, in the setting. It is equally appropriate to shorten the session and ensure the client feels safe before moving forward with their day. Neurodivergent clients often benefit from journaling, creating art, or recording a video to document the experience and explore insights that emerged, for their own reference. These can be effective ways to deepen their experience of safely moving through dysregulation, and of encoding it in memory. Providing clients with creative ways to encode and retain their therapeutic experience is an accessibility feature of NAP.

Autistic burnout

A neurodivergent child who experiences frequent limbic activation becomes a neurodivergent adult who is familiar with the experience of *autistic burnout.* This is a seriously disabling state of mental and physical depletion that simply cannot be ignored by the individual and must not be ignored by family and friends. Autistic burnout is more than dysregulation. It is a mental health crisis that requires recognition and appropriate care, that occurs uniquely in the neurodivergent population, and that is poorly researched and sparsely documented in the extant literature. Autistic burnout is described by lived experts as a "highly debilitating condition characterized by exhaustion, withdrawal, executive functioning problems, and generally reduced functioning, with increased manifestation of autistic traits – and distinct from depression and non-autistic burnout" (Higgins et al., 2021, p. 2356). Raymaker et al. (2020, p. 132) emphasised the distinction between autistic burnout and occupational burnout, proposing the following definition:

> *Autistic burnout is a syndrome conceptualised as resulting from chronic life stress and a mismatch of expectations and abilities without adequate supports. It is characterised by pervasive, long-term (typically 3+ months) exhaustion, loss of function and reduced tolerance to stimulus.*

Autistic individuals experiencing burnout report feeling chronically exhausted, often from the daily demands of navigating multiple sensory challenges and social interactions in public spaces. For many, the stress of constant masking depletes energy, triggers defence mechanisms, and precipitates a state of shutdown that requires complete physical and emotional withdrawal. The signs and symptoms of autistic burnout include a deep and prolonged exhaustion that autistic clients may describe as total depletion of their internal resources: physical, mental, social, and emotional (Raymaker et al., 2020). Clients describe a pervasive loss of executive functioning capacity; planning, recalling, organizing, time management, and decision-making are unavailable, disrupting work, education, parenting, and even the ability to take basic care of oneself. They also report difficulty with listening and speaking; avoidance of social contact; a compelling need for quiet, dark, and scent-free environments; inability to shop, cook, or eat; aversion to the executive functioning demands and sensory aspects of personal hygiene; and incapacity to care for pets, elders, or children. Some individuals experience an increase in neurological symptoms such as tics, seizures, or compulsive behaviours associated with autistic burnout, which may or may not be observable in the therapy room.

The struggle to keep pace with increased stress and compounding factors such as those described above stretches, and will eventually exceed, most autistic individual's executive functioning capacity, if relief is not provided. The individual's usual daily chores and responsibilities – cooking and feeding themselves and their family, making and keeping appointments, caring for young children or elders, commuting to work, attending to pets – begin to feel overwhelming. They may report unusual difficulty planning and prioritising, making choices or decisions, or maintaining their usual degree of order. They may lose keys or wallets, forget important dates and details, or miss appointments. In this compromised state of mental functioning, one's capacity for self-soothing, creativity, relational satisfaction, shared emotion, and all kinds of learning, is curtailed. Self-aware individuals recognise these functional difficulties as signs their capacity for executive functioning is over-stretched and change is needed, and without delay. This may take the form of pausing to reassess the situation, re-prioritising, asking a carefully chosen individual for help, or temporarily delegating some responsibilities to others. It may include an increase in self-care, adjustment of dietary, exercise, meditation or sleep habits, or a review of medication, if applicable. Healthy individuals interpret the physical, emotional, and psychological signs of overwhelm as important information, and make adjustments before their prefrontal cortex shuts down and their limbic system takes control, in a valiant (but often unnecessary) attempt to save their lives! Less healthy or less self-aware individuals are inclined to ignore the signs, double down, push through, self-isolate, self-medicate, or similar, ironically increasing the likelihood of completely overwhelming their thinking brain, rather than supporting themselves in intentional, simple, self-compassionate ways.

Currently, much of the available understanding and support for individuals experiencing autistic burnout comes from the online autistic community, and from practice-based evidence from clinicians and settings providing NAP. Individuals with lived experience attribute it to the multiple, ever-changing, sensory, and social demands of school, work, and home – in tandem with the absence of support, space, or time autistic people need to recharge their internal batteries, daily. The all-consuming experience of autistic burnout was described by one individual as follows:

> In autistic burnout, I am like a mirror that shatters in all directions at once. The image I had of myself and the world around me is suddenly all in pieces and crashing down around me. I can't catch the pieces no matter how hard I work, and I just want to curl up on the floor, cover my eyes and ears, and never move again.

Autistic individuals experiencing burnout may need practical support to withdraw from work demands and family obligations, for as long as it takes to recover their sense of inner balance and safety. Importantly, autistic burnout impacts executive functioning, reducing the individuals' capacity for decision-making and sometimes calling on psychotherapists to take an unusually directive role in identifying what is happening, and activating supports.

Neurodivergent clients who are poorly supported at home may need professional care for autistic burnout, but this option should be exercised very cautiously, if at all. Autistic advocates highlight that hospitalization is rarely the best approach to burnout because of the aversive sensory environment of hospitals and clinics, alongside the risk of misdiagnosis and inappropriate medical treatment. Many neurodivergent individuals, and particularly those who identify as female, have been misdiagnosed (and medically treated) for serious psychiatric diagnoses including Borderline Personality Disorder (BPD) and Schizoaffective Disorder, when in fact they were experiencing autistic burnout (Arnold et al., 2023), and urgently needed a prolonged period of time alone, with ample rest, darkness, and quiet. This is important for clinicians to understand because psychotherapists are often responsible for informed and effective advocacy, in times when clients are overwhelmed and unable to speak for themselves.

An episode of autistic burnout motivates some individuals to request psychotherapy, hoping to gather information about what happened, and to explore whether and how they can avoid experiencing it again. Clear, accurate information is often very reassuring to autistic individuals, many of whom draw support from the cognitive domain before the emotional. However, autistic individuals in burnout also need recognition, validation, and support for their emotional experience. As previously mentioned, requesting psychotherapy is often a departure from their default or preferred approach to problem-solving, for autistic individuals. In my clinical experience, many autistic individuals are understandably cautious of healthcare professionals, with or without the proverbial "white coat", based on their own previous negative experiences.

Not uncommonly, the crash into autistic burnout seems to the individual to have occurred quite suddenly, taking them (and sometimes also their family or colleagues) by surprise. Although it has often been building for some time, reduced interoceptive awareness has often resulted in the individual missing the internal signs, sometimes throughout their life to date. For this reason, autistic individuals within my practice who experience prolonged or severe autistic burnout are rarely encouraged to return to their pre-burnout level of functioning; rather, they are supported to understand their sensory experience, and to reassess their values and goals alongside a fresh and deeper commitment to self-awareness, self-care, and self-preservation.

Autism and self-awareness

While it has been proposed that reduced awareness of self and others is a feature of autism (Baron-Cohen, 2008), it is also argued that the existence of masking as a coping mechanism effectively challenges this contention (Radulski, 2022); neurodivergent individuals would not mask if they were completely unaware of the differences between their ways of being and those of neurotypicals. While it seems likely that degrees of self-awareness differ between neurodivergent individuals as between neurotypicals, many autistic individuals endorse the distressing sensation of suddenly feeling overwhelmed and somewhat sabotaged by their emotions, in response to *sensory overload*. Clients report that this happens "out of nowhere"; it seems to creep up and pounce like an alley cat, claws spread wide! Hyposensitive interoception, along with the rapidity and intensity with which many neurodivergent individuals become dysregulated makes it challenging for them to notice the early signs and redirect the downward spiral; self-awareness is therefore an important area for neurodivergent individuals to explore in therapy.

Most people find it challenging to establish or maintain self-regulation when their interoceptive systems are conveying messages of fatigue, hunger, or physical discomfort; these sensations must be prioritized. In conditions that produce a fear response, whether those conditions exist outside or inside the individual, self-awareness enables people to intentionally act to restore balance – often by using their senses to do a "reality check" on the real or perceived threat. Sensations of fear in the body (tightness in the throat or chest, sweaty or clammy skin) call on the person to pause and investigate whether there is really a lion in the bush, or whether it has been placed there (very convincingly) by their own imagination! This is an important awareness in

NAP because many neurodivergent individuals have difficulty intentionally increasing self-awareness, while neurotypicals often learn to do so with relative ease. As previously noted, neurodivergent individuals may miss internal "early warning signs" of dysregulation. Subtle internal messages such as vague tightness in the throat, or a slight sensation of heat in the hands, may not register consciously for neurodivergent individuals, or may be obscured by hyperfocus elsewhere, in that moment. Vague internal sensations often carry important messages however, which usually intensify gradually until attention is paid. By the time they are noticeable, however, the autistic/neurodivergent individual may be significantly dysregulated, and beyond the possibility of quick or easy self-regulation.

Reduced self-awareness combined with hyperfocus results in significant challenges for neurodivergent children when the sensory demands of the classroom or chaos of the schoolyard exceed their capacity to self-regulate. Most school boards have yet to recognize the nexus between neurodivergent kids' deep focus, difficulty with shifting attention, and neurologically determined sensory needs. Autistic kids are often resourceful, creative thinkers, and many develop coping mechanisms to manage their own dysregulation, not all of which meet with the approval of school systems. Such coping mechanisms may include rapidly exiting an overwhelming situation, self-isolating, seeking deep pressure through physical altercations with peers or adults, climbing trees, or self-harming. Sadly, it is not unusual to meet a neurodivergent young adult who graduated from high school with good grades, but also carried home a backpack filled with anger, sadness, and unresolved school-based trauma. Many experienced bullying and exclusion by peers and adults, and discriminatory policies throughout their school years, and seek therapy to explore the pain, grieve the loss of opportunity, and resolve the resultant shame. These individuals often benefit from recognition and validation of their unique sensory needs, hyperfocus and reduced self-awareness, and confirmation that their suffering would have been significantly reduced or prevented if their neurotype had been recognized by the adults who were responsible for their protection and education.

Supportive sensory experience is a cornerstone of NAP; autistic/neurodivergent individuals are offered a positive relational experience which intentionally centres their unique sensory profile. The goals, pace, and process of therapy are framed accordingly, with the following intentions made explicit:

1.   to highlight the importance of understanding and utilizing sensory processing in establishing and maintaining mental health;
2.   to invite conversations about knowing, expressing, and meeting one's sensory needs within relationships and to identify how/if the client is currently aware of and attending to these;

3. to provide direct experience of the positive impact of sensory support on verbal and non-verbal communication;
4. to assemble an individualized set of effective sensory-based tools and permission for self-care; and
5. to prioritize sensory supports to address exhaustion, or to prevent/treat autistic burnout.

In NAP, a sensory-supportive therapeutic environment is intentionally provided, where the neurodivergent client can learn to pay attention to their sensory experience, experiment with trusting the messages received through those channels, and settle more comfortably within their own mind and body – recognizing the experiences of safety and belonging that are available here. Simultaneously, a secure attachment relationship is offered, within which the client is supported to identify and articulate their needs and desires, increase their capacity for trust, receive unconditional acceptance and positive regard, and experience their positive impact on another person. The blend of *attachment-based therapy within a sensory-supportive environment* is the foundational framework for NAP.

Integrating sensory processing into the therapeutic alliance

The intensity, quality and depth of an individual's sensory experiences are determined by their *sensory profile*. If this concept and language is unfamiliar, psychotherapists can explore their own sensory profile and bring their own sensory preferences and aversions to awareness, before attempting to work with clients in this way. Accessible psychometric tools such as the Adult and Adolescent Sensory Assessment (AASA) may be used to self-examine and reflect, in preparation for the practical exercise of increasing ones' own awareness and adapting the therapeutic environment to meet the needs of neurodivergent clients.

Aside from creating an accessible, safe, and welcoming environment, providing a sensory-supportive therapeutic space reduces the risk of sensory-based microaggressions toward neurodivergent individuals in therapy. Sue (2010, p. xvi) defines microaggressions as "commonplace verbal, behavioural, or environmental slights, whether intentional or unintentional, that communicate hostile, derogatory, or negative attitudes toward stigmatized or culturally marginalized groups". Additionally, the perpetrator of a microaggression remains unaware that they have inadvertently behaved in a way that threatens or demeans a marginalized individual (Sue & Spanierman, 2020). Irrespective of the therapeutic modalities in which a therapist practices, every client brings their sensory profile into the room, and in neurodiversity-affirming practice it is recognized, welcomed, and employed as a valuable resource within the therapeutic alliance.

Many neurodivergent individuals have developed unique and creative ways to meet their sensory needs in their own homes, and much is learned about the supports an individual requires by listening to what they already provide for themselves in their private spaces. It is also important to explore with these individuals whether and how their sensory needs are recognized and met by those with whom they live, work, or study – or conversely, are ignored or treated as inconveniences. This topic should be revisited periodically throughout the course of therapy, with the intentions of encouraging the client to recognize the critical role of sensory processing in attaining/maintaining their own mental health, empowering them to attend to it as a daily basic need (like food, sleep, and shelter), to enhance their wellbeing and prevent autistic burnout, and to increase their fluency in self-advocacy when needed.

Sensory-based adaptations will either enhance the therapeutic experience or have neutral effect on neurotypical clients, while increasing accessibility for neurodivergent clients. They provide a plug for the ongoing drain of sensory-based energy, ideally making a small pool of energy available to the individual for the therapeutic process. When successful, this little pool will be spring fed, becoming a renewable resource that the client will draw upon when needed, far beyond therapy. Ideally, their therapeutic experience gives neurodivergent clients permission and encouragement to reflect on how they might adapt their own homes and workplaces to conserve their energy by working with rather than against their own sensory profile, and to advocate for sensory-based adaptations to schools, workplaces, healthcare facilities, and elsewhere. Sensory-supportive environments quieten "noise", particularly auditory and visual, providing an experience of spaciousness, attentiveness, and personal safety, for those who need it, while detracting nothing from the experience of those who do not.

Since every individual has a unique sensory profile, it is clinically appropriate to provide a unique sensory environment for each client in therapy. A welcoming space for neurodivergent clients is created by reflecting on what is known about the effects of physical space on mental health, alongside what is known about the specific client's neurological profile. Holding all of this, alongside awareness of the high probability that a neurodivergent client is bringing a trauma history to therapy, we arrange the waiting area and therapy room and plan our sessions accordingly.

Offering psychotherapy to neurodivergent clients in a sensory environment they find intolerable is not only discriminatory. It is also a waste of resources, reminiscent of a time when a building that could only be accessed by a staircase was unrecognized as inaccessible to individuals who use wheelchairs for mobility. Clearly, if a client cannot access psychotherapy because they experience the sensory environment as aversive, immediate change to the environment is indicated, along with gratitude to the client for articulating their needs, and a genuine apology for the microaggression. Not every therapist is freely to create or adapt their own therapy environment; many work in shared space within agencies and educational/healthcare institutions and have limited flexibility with design or adaptation. In all such settings, however, there are also neurodivergent staff, whose daily sensory experience depletes and exhausts them significantly more than their neurotypical colleagues, and who may not yet be ready to disclose or self-advocate. Creating a sensory-supportive environment in which to provide therapy to neurodivergent clients will also meet the needs of neurodivergent staff; it is an accessibility requirement, and should be prioritized accordingly in resource allocation, in all public settings.

Chapter 9 provides practical, sensory-based adaptations to guide the preparation of a therapeutic environment that will be accessible to most autistic/neurodivergent individuals, even without advance knowledge of the client's unique sensory profile.

Sample therapeutic questions on sensory processing and self-awareness

1. Do you identify as a highly sensitive person? Tell me about your own sensory profile. Are you especially sensitive to certain sensory experiences, such as particular smells or sounds? How does this impact you personally, or your relationships with others?

2. Tell me about a time in childhood when you felt like your parents/caregivers really understood your sensory needs. Tell me about a time when you felt as if your sensory profile was not understood by parents/caregivers. Why do you think this occurred? What do you wish the adults had known, or done differently, at that time?

3. Have you ever lost a job, or had to move home or school, because of sensory issues? Please tell me about that experience.

4. What do you need me/us to do or not do, to ensure that your sensory needs are integrated and welcomed within your therapeutic experience?

5. How often do you sit and listen to the sounds from inside your own body? Are there some sounds you find especially intriguing or entertaining? Are there any that you dislike or find worrisome?

6. How often do you eat with other people? Are you familiar with misophonia, and is it part of your own sensory profile? How do you manage it? Is there anything you really want to do that is prevented by misophonia?

7. Tell me about the animals in your life. In what ways do your pets provide sensory support?

8. When you think about your elementary school days, what sounds and smells come to mind? Were these pleasant or unpleasant experiences, and how much control did you have over them, on a day-to-day basis?

References

American Psychiatric Association. (2022). Diagnostic and statistical manual of mental disorders (5th ed., text rev.). https://doi.org/10.1176/appi.books.9780890425787

Arnold, S. R., Higgins, J. M., Weise, J., Desai, A., Pellicano, E., & Trollor, J. N. (2023). Confirming the nature of autistic burnout. *Autism, 20*(7), 1906–1918.

Aron, E. N. (2013). *The highly sensitive person: How to thrive when the world overwhelms you.* Kensington Publishing.

Ayres, A. J. (1972). Improving academic scores through sensory integration. *Journal of Learning Disabilities, 5*(6), 338–343.

Baron-Cohen, S. (2008). *Autism and Asperger syndrome.* OUP Oxford.

Barrett, A. C. (2020). *Symptom presentation of children with Autism spectrum disorder after adverse childhood experiences.* University of California.

Cain, S. (2013). *Quiet: The power of introverts in a world that can't stop talking.* Crown.

Grassmann, H., Stupiggia, M., & Porges, S. W. (2023). The science of embodiment: Trauma, body, and relationship. *International Body Psychotherapy Journal, 22*(1), 149.

Greenberg, L. S. (2004). Emotion–focused therapy. *Clinical Psychology & Psychotherapy: An International Journal of Theory & Practice, 11*(1), 3–16.

Higgins, J. M., Arnold, S. R., Weise, J., Pellicano, E., & Trollor, J. N. (2021). Defining autistic burnout through experts by lived experience: Grounded Delphi method investigating# AutisticBurnout. *Autism, 25*(8), 2356–2369.

Jackson-Perry, D., Rosqvist, H. B., Annable, J. L., & Kourti, M. (2020). Sensory strangers: Travels in normate sensory worlds. In H. Rosqvist, N. Chown, & A. Stenning (Eds.), *Neurodiversity studies; a new critical paradigm.* (pp. 125–149). Routledge.

Kilroy, E., Aziz-Zadeh, L., & Cermak, S. (2019). Ayres theories of autism and sensory integration revisited: What contemporary neuroscience has to say. *Brain Sciences, 9*(3), 68–88.

Kumar, S., Tansley-Hancock, O., Sedley, W., Winston, J. S., Callaghan, M. F., Allen, M., Cope, T. E., Gander, P. E., Bamiou, D. E., & Griffiths, T. D. (2017). The brain basis for misophonia. *Current Biology, 27*(4), 527–533. https://doi.org/10.1016/J.CUB.2016.12.048

Levine, K. (2016). Replays: A therapeutic approach for children with Autism Spectrum Disorder. In A. A. Drewes & C. E. Schaefer (Eds.), *Play therapy in middle childhood* (pp. 275–290). American Psychological Association.

Levine, P. A., Blakeslee, A., & Sylvae, J. (2018). Reintegrating fragmentation of the primitive self: Discussion of "somatic experiencing"." *Psychoanalytic Dialogues, 28*(5), 620–628.

Machingura, T., & Lloyd, C. (2017). Sensory approaches in mental health: Contemporary occupation-based practice or a redundant medical approach? *International Journal of Therapy and Rehabilitation, 24*(5), 189. https://doi.org/10.12968/IJTR.2017.24.9.373

Morgan, H. (2019). Connections between sensory sensitivities in Autism; The importance of sensory friendly environments for accessibility and increased quality of life for the neurodivergent autistic minority. *PSU McNair Scholars Online Journal, 13*(1), 1.

Nerenberg, J. (2020). *Divergent mind: Thriving in a world that wasn't designed for you.* HarperOne.

Nesin-Perna, S. (2023). *The interaction of mental health and executive function among neurodiverse University students* [Doctoral Dissertation]. University of Massachusetts Lowell.

Parham, L. D., & Crickmore, D. (2022). *Expanding sensory awareness. Intellectual disabilities-E-book: Toward inclusion* (Vol. 231). Elsevier Health Sciences.

Phillips, A. (2010). *On balance.* Farrar, Straus and Giroux.

Porges, S. W., & Dana, D. (2018). *Clinical applications of the polyvagal theory: The emergence of polyvagal-informed therapies (Norton series on interpersonal neurobiology).* WW Norton & Company.

Radulski, E. M. (2022). Conceptualising autistic masking, camouflaging, and neurotypical privilege: Towards a minority group model of neurodiversity. *Human Development, 66*(2), 113–127.

Randell, E., Wright, M., Milosevic, S., Gillespie, D., Brookes-Howell, L., Busse-Morris, M., Hastings, R., Maboshe, W., Williams-Thomas, R., Mills, L., Romeo, R., Yaziji, N., McKigney, A. M., Ahuja, A., Warren, G., Glarou, E., Delport, S., & McNamara, R. (2022). Sensory integration therapy for children with autism and sensory processing difficulties: The SenITA RCT. *Health Technology Assessment, 26*(29), 2. https://doi.org/10.3310/TQGE0020

Raymaker, D. M., Teo, A. R., Steckler, N. A., Lentz, B., Scharer, M., Delos Santos, A., Kapp, S. K., Hunter, M., Joyce, A., & Nicolaidis, C. (2020). "Having all of your internal resources exhausted beyond measure and being left with no clean-up crew": Defining autistic burnout. *Autism in Adulthood: Challenges and Management, 2*(2), 132–143. https://doi.org/10.1089/AUT.2019.0079

Shanker, S. (2010). Self-regulation: Calm, alert, and learning. *Education Canada, 50*(3), 4–7.

Sue, D. W. (2010). *Microaggressions in everyday life: Race, gender, and sexual orientation.* John Wiley & Sons, Inc.

Sue, D. W., & Spanierman, L. (2020). *Microaggressions in everyday life.* John Wiley & Sons.

Sutton, D., Wilson, M., Van Kessel, K., & Vanderpyl, J. (2013). Optimizing arousal to manage aggression: A pilot study of sensory modulation. *International Journal of Mental Health Nursing, 22*(6), 500–511. https://doi.org/10.1111/INM.12010

Communication and neurodivergence

The ability to be understood and to exchange information with other human beings is typically taken for granted by neurotypical individuals; not so for neurodivergent people, who often struggle with the impacts of unsatisfactory communication exchanges, across neurotypes. This chapter highlights the mental health impacts of the social communication and social interaction experiences of autistic individuals, with the goals of facilitating therapeutic conversations and informing advocacy. This chapter supports informal observation and assessment of the communication features of autism/neurodivergence, and explores their relational impacts within the dominant culture. Clinical strategies that reconcile autistic and allistic communication within NAP are provided in Chapter 9.

Chapter 6 responds to the following clinical questions:

1. What is the role of communication in *attachment relationships*?
2. What are some notable features of communication exchanges between individuals with different neurotypes?
3. How can a neurotypical therapist adjust communication to provide a neurodiversity-affirming therapeutic experience?
4. What is the relevance of DSM-5 (American Psychiatric Association, 2022) communication-related diagnostic criteria to the process of psychotherapy with autistic clients?

Communication happens in the space between people (Hobson et al., 2022), and, ideally, facilitates mutual understanding and shared experiences. Gutstein (2009) articulated that mutually satisfying communication involves combining something from one person with something from another, with the shared anticipation that something new and unique (and possibly better than either idea alone) will emerge.

In psychotherapy, autistic individuals often express confusion, frustration, and even sadness about their experiences of communication in important relationships with allistic (non-autistic) or other neurodivergent individuals. In the

DOI: 10.4324/9781003430476-6

contexts of personal and professional relationships, and equally within quick, casual interactions, autistic individuals regularly describe interactions with neurotypicals that have felt puzzling, incomplete, or otherwise enigmatic. Clients describe a vague sense that the other person seems to have had an opportunity to review the "rules" for the interaction, or had advance notice of the outcome, while they did not have that same opportunity. This sensation regularly elicits uncomfortable feelings and thoughts associated with being at a disadvantage in social life. Clients describe the requirement to spread their attention so thinly as to make it impossible to keep pace with the content of an interaction; of getting stuck on a detail and missing what followed; of feeling oneself detaching from the interaction and watching oneself slipping into silence. Autistic clients frequently express that there is something mysterious about how neurotypical people communicate. Confusion is expressed around neurotypical social skills, which include generating and participating in "small talk"; discerning and joining the flow of a group conversation; and interpreting the meaning conveyed by facial expressions and body gestures. The experience of feeling partially or completely excluded from social life is a familiar and painful experience for many autistic individuals whose lives intersect regularly with neurotypicals at home or elsewhere. Selective (or situational) mutism – a sudden inability to speak in a specific setting or situation – is a common manifestation of social anxiety in autistic individuals and is explored in detail later in this chapter.

Autistic clients have noted in therapy that the more meaningful or important a relationship is to them, the more complex the communicative demands and expectations seem to be. This perception understandably increases anxiety; the higher the value a relationship has for an individual, the higher the stakes if communication breaks down. These individuals also report frustration with the unwritten, complex, and ever-changing rules of verbal and non-verbal communication, or with missing information that was conveyed within a cacophony of multiple channels of communication operating simultaneously. Such moments occur daily for autistic individuals, in social contexts such as classrooms, clinical settings, shopping malls and restaurants, exacerbating the anxiety that is already so prevalent in this population.

Some autistic individuals report that a conversation with one other person is enough to trigger a compensatory mechanism which may take the form of withdrawal from the interaction or may alternatively manifest as increased volume and/or hyper-verbalizing. Such compensations are regularly misinterpreted by neurotypicals as attempts to dominate the conversation, or to control the outcome. They attest to the significant effort required by the autistic individual to filter extraneous visual and auditory input from the environment, while simultaneously attending to the speaker's voice, facial expressions, and somatic gestures. For many autistic individuals, expanding this experience to situations where multiple voices are speaking, such as a holiday meal, classroom, or team meeting, demands an inordinate expenditure of energy, requiring intentional, ongoing self-care during the experience and recovery time and space, afterward.

Intimate partnerships between individuals of different neurotypes are frequently recognized by the partners only after one or more of their children receives a diagnosis of autism/ADHD. It is particularly important for couples' therapists to recognize that such pairs often need to work harder (or differently) than those with similar neurotypes, to establish and maintain ongoing, mutually satisfying communication. In the best of such partnerships, this hard work is offset by rich and unique relational experiences, bringing out the best in both individuals and creating an environment of mutual appreciation and respect. When this occurs, such partners can challenge neuronormativity in the dominant culture, by openly celebrating neurodiversity within their family and setting the stage for secure attachment relationships and accordingly robust mental health.

Neurodivergent adults may seek diagnosis or not; many prefer to explore their neurodivergent identity in therapy without incurring the expense and stress associated with the diagnostic process. Not infrequently, neurodivergent adults experience significant relief in response to their increased self-understanding, having struggled with varying degrees of social discomfort, relational dissatisfaction, and difficulties with "fitting in" throughout their lives, with neither a plausible explanation nor appropriate supports. Relief is a common response to receiving an adult diagnosis, as it is to recognizing one's own neurodivergence. Adults in this situation may experience anger, sadness, frustration, or denial, sometimes (and not always) intertwined with relief, vindication, or self-acceptance. Given this melange, some late-diagnosed adults benefit from acknowledging and attending to grief and loss in therapy, while others will need their therapist to join in celebrating their newly identified neurodivergence!

Challenging neuronormativity

When they are well, autistic individuals are direct and honest communicators who are appreciated and valued by colleagues, friends and partners for the precision, clarity, insight, and authenticity with which they communicate (De Clercq et al., 2019). Often, the highly creative problem solving, unique sense of humour, and unshakeable commitment to fairness and justice that autistic individuals offer, significantly enhance their own and others' experiences of important relationships and preferred activities. Autistic individuals frequently speak up when they perceive injustice or discrimination, rather than remaining silent out of concern about the opinions of others. Hartman et al. (2023) demonstrated that in the workplace, autistic individuals are less impacted than neurotypicals by the so-called "bystander effect", where neurotypicals may ignore wrongdoing that they witness while in a group of colleagues or peers. Healthy, well-rested autistic individuals are independent thinkers and truth tellers; they often detect patterns in apparent chaos, and are not afraid to "call bullshit" when indicated! Indeed, it is my belief that the little boy who proclaimed the truth loudly and clearly in the children's story "The Emperor's New Clothes" was certainly autistic. Unaffected by the web of secrets and lies around him, he saw clearly that the emperor was completely naked, and his brave articulation of that truth liberated the townspeople from years of oppression, silencing, and collusion: an autistic triumph, undoubtedly!

Expressive communication is so much more than words. Throughout history, neurodivergent artists and musicians have communicated their intense sensory experience and unique perspectives through extraordinary works of art and music, enriching others' experience accordingly. The unique perspectives and independent and generative thinking of neurodivergent individuals drive invention and advance research worldwide. Parents of recently diagnosed autistic children are sometimes interested in hearing the names of notable historical figures who are believed (or known) to have been autistic (James, 2005). Those names include scientists (Albert Einstein and Isaac Newton), composers (Ludwig van Beethoven and Wolfgang Mozart), inventors (Henry Ford and Benjamin Franklin), and renowned psychiatrist/psychotherapist Carl Jung. They also include many currently prominent figures such as entrepreneurs Bill Gates and Elon Musk, musicians John Denver and James Taylor, surfer Clay Marzo, and actor Dan Aykroyd. On the other hand, it is important to note that although such information may encourage neurotypical parents who are concerned about their autistic child's future, many autistic advocates have expressed frustration with the implication that these exceptional individuals are representative of all neurodivergent people. There is a range of cognitive ability among the neurodivergent population, just as there is in the neurotypical. Billeiter and Froiland (2023) highlighted that determining the diversity of intelligence among autistic people has implications for research, clinical practice, and neurological understanding; the same can of course be said about the neurotypical population. Additionally, psychotherapists recognize that unique and impressive artistic contributions often emerge from an individual's suffering, or their struggle for acceptance and belonging within the dominant culture; this narrative resonates for many autistic individuals. Notwithstanding the above, the final word on this topic must go to the iconic autistic individual who recently informed me (with a giggle) that "I don't have the name-in-the-history-books kind of autism. I have the notice-every-tiny-detail-and-find-it-impossible-to-filter-any-of-it-out, kind of autism!"

While recognizing and valuing the many strengths that neurodivergent individuals bring to relationships (and therefore, to the therapeutic alliance), psychotherapists providing NAP also recognize the communication-related challenges that DSM-5 (American Psychiatric Association, 2022) describes as a central diagnostic criterion for autism. The extent to which these features are apparent, and their relational impact, varies greatly, as does the degree to which they are experienced as impediments to quality of life by the individual and those who matter in their world. It is toward the communication-related features and their potential impacts on autistic mental health that we now turn.

Human communication, the verbal and non-verbal behaviour by which humans share thoughts, ideas, opinions, emotions, and imaginings – indeed any element of their mental activity they wish to share – is foundational to the quality of their relational experience. From birth, optimal psychological development and infant mental health require regular, easeful interactions with a caring adult; babies that receive interested, encouraging responses to their early communicative attempts are thus reinforced to make incremental efforts to continue to engage by communicating, facilitating healthy development (Ilyka et al., 2021). Conversely, in the absence of an effective communication system between infants and their parents, the child's developmental potential is inevitably curtailed (Doove et al., 2021). Well-rested, typically developing human babies cannot resist invitations from loving parents and caregivers to interact, and regularly initiate such interactions themselves. Once an interaction begins, typically developing babies continue to strive to keep the adult engaged by gazing, smiling, and eventually vocalizing. In response, adults naturally imitate and enhance each sound, and respond to the infant's changing facial expressions, as they interact within the safe container of their emergent attachment relationship (Karakaş & Dağlı, 2019). Mutually satisfying communication is integral to healthy relationships. Although regular glitches and breakdowns in communication inevitably occur, the sustainability of a relationship is often apparent in the capacity and willingness of the individuals involved to recognize communication rupture, large or small, and to take intentional, reparative action when necessary.

Communication and attachment relationships

Humans are born fully dependent, and their survival depends upon establishing a functional, reciprocal communication system with their carers (Fogel, 1993; Gutstein, 2000). The communication feedback loop between parents and babies is inextricably linked to brain development; early parent-child interactions establish neurological pathways which largely determine the quality of the attachment relationship between the two (Parsons et al., 2010; Ulmer-Yaniv et al., 2022). Attachment relationships across the lifespan mirror the infant's experience within those early interactions (Rees, 2007), often reflecting the quality of the communication between them and their primary attachment figures (Bowlby, 1979; Main, 1996).

Interpersonal communication is a central element of rich life experience; humans demonstrate the desire for communication with others from before they are born to the end of their conscious lives. With rudimentary communication skills and abilities, newborn babies convey sufficient information to adults to get their needs for love, food, comfort, and social interaction met, remarkably effectively. Every communicative exchange between parent and baby in the first 18 months refines the parent-child feedback loop, facilitating the development of secure attachment while also ensuring the baby's needs are met, providing incremental degrees of mutual satisfaction for both people, and fostering a sense of personal agency within the baby. Parent-child communication becomes a familiar dance, the well-known steps of which must change at the other end of the story. The well-established dance between a parent and child shifts and dissolves, in the transition from life to death. While accompanying my dad through the last days of his life, a moment occurred where I became suddenly aware that our communication dance had ended, some indeterminate time before. Dad was still alive, but an unfamiliar and irreversible quietness had softly entered the space between us. In the same moment I realized it had ended, the invaluable gift of the unique communication dance between my father and I became clearer than ever before, allowing gratitude to arrive and grieving to begin. Such is the profound importance of communication between people in attachment relationships, across the lifespan, and beyond.

Verbal and non-verbal communication

Verbal communication – the exchange of words – is a somewhat messy cacophony by which humans attempt to share their inner worlds with one another. However, words are just one element of human communication. It is sometimes proposed that the impact of words is minimal; that our authentic communication is non-verbal, consisting of gestures and facial expressions over which we have varying degrees of control. In most social contexts, non-verbal communication is interpreted (and responded to) intertwined with verbal, predisposing us to all sorts of unhelpful and unproductive interactions. At the same time, it is important to recognize that although human communication is often complicated, and vulnerable to misinterpretation, in the big picture, humans generally manage to communicate with one another well enough to create safety, facilitate connection, share ideas, and confide aspirations, and even at times to encourage, inspire and delight one another. This truly matters, not only to the survival of the species, but also to safeguard against silencing ourselves and one another, for fear of offending, or of mockery or disregard by other people.

Mehrabian (1972) and Mehrabian and Ferris (1967) posited that when an individual's verbal and nonverbal communication appear incongruous to an observer, the non-verbal component is significantly more reliable than the verbal. Distilled, Mehrabian's findings were that 93% of communication is non-verbal and only 7% is verbal, in moments when verbal and non-verbal communication seem misaligned. Lapakko (2007) extrapolated that in moments of high emotion (of which psychotherapy is often one) the non-verbal component of communication should be considered the more accurate in inferring meaning. While Mehrabian's 93:7 ratio is still conventional wisdom, it is laced with neuronormative presuppositions. My clinical experience suggests that although it may be somewhat plausible in situations where the communicators and the observer all have the same neurotype, it is an unhelpful framework when considering cross-neurotype communication. Since the central concern in NAP is establishing and sustaining the therapeutic alliance when client and therapist have different neurotypes, a postmodern perspective of communication as an emergent, dynamic process that is co-created between people, is more helpful. Through this lens, the direction and outcomes of interpersonal communication depend heavily on context; on invisible or unnamed elements such as the balance of power, the relative safety of the environment, and the histories, expectations and goals of speaker and listener. In wider society, the outcomes of interpersonal communication may be influenced by observable elements such as hand and body movements, facial expressions, and cosmetic forms of self-expression including clothing, hairstyle, piercing, and tattoos. Observable elements of self-presentation are also non-verbal elements of communication, and therefore open to (mis)interpretation in wider society – it is clearly important that this phenomenon is not reflected within the cross-neurotype therapeutic alliance.

Therapist self-awareness becomes increasingly imperative as awareness and appreciation of neurodiversity increases. Psychotherapists are professional listeners, creators, and holders of healing spaces where individuals can be their authentic selves. As such, it is essential that we work from a place of awareness, dynamically identifying and intentionally releasing any inclination to interpret a client's non-verbal communication through a neuronormative cultural lens. Especially when working with neurodivergent individuals, replacing such interpretation with continued observation, respectful curiosity, and unconditional acceptance, is a significantly clearer pathway to effective cross-cultural communication between different neurotypes.

Autistic communication and self-expression

As outlined in Chapter 2, the diagnostic criteria for autism include: "persistent deficits in social communication and social interaction" (DSM-5, American Psychiatric Association, 2022). Such "deficits" must be observed in social-emotional reciprocity, in non-verbal communication, and in the individual's capacity for developing and maintaining relationships. It is very apparent that, when viewed through a neuronormative lens, a diagnosis of autism suggests significantly impacted social communication. This deficit-laden perspective of autistic communication is problematic for many neurodivergent individuals, who experience it as overgeneralized, pathologizing, and patronizing. Neurodivergent advocates regularly and legitimately object to the notion that autistic communication, which differs among individuals with as much variance as neurotypical communication, is viewed by diagnosticians as unilaterally in deficit. Autistic advocates highlight that although they often communicate at a different pace than neurotypicals, use distinctive vocabulary or speak with a tone, rhythm or volume that differs from the neurotypical norm, none of these features necessarily constitute a deficit; they are differences, and if they are problematic in some circles, it is neuronormativity that renders them so.

Verbal communication and language

Much has been written about the difficulties autistic/neurodivergent individuals encounter in back-and-forth verbal exchanges with neurotypicals. Clients in my practice regularly report an uncomfortable feeling, as if they are interrupting other people or others are interrupting them, within conversations – along with a unilateral sense of responsibility for their own discomfort. A well-recognized (if poorly understood) feature of autistic verbal communication is observable in the enthusiasm with which autistic individuals communicate about their personal interests or areas of expertise. Many autistic individuals enjoy "intense and focused interest in a narrow range of subjects" (Klin et al., 2007), or in a specific and often highly specialized area of study (Harrop et al., 2019, p. 64). highlighted that personal interests at the intensity and depth to which autistic individuals engage with them, often represent significant areas of ability and expertise. Frequently, autistic adults have been exploring and studying their areas of expertise since childhood, and have organized their career, social, or recreational activities accordingly. Individuals whose areas of expertise have been rejected or ridiculed by neurotypicals often suffer greatly for want of welcoming opportunities to discuss, explore, and share them with other people.

Diagnostically, personal interests are considered a "subcategory of restricted and repetitive behaviors that occur commonly in individuals with autism spectrum disorder" (Harrop et al., 2019, p. 63). From a neurodiversity viewpoint, this is controversial, and is experienced by many autistic adults as pathologizing and demeaning. Many autistic people have had difficulty finding neurotypicals who have the capacity for hyperfocus that is required to engage as deeply and for such lengthy periods as they can and do, with their particular interests. Consequently, this is a common area for communicative rupture between neurotypes; autistic adults may initially be reluctant to share their area of interest in psychotherapy, especially if they have a history of being silenced or reprimanded for doing so in neuronormative environments. However, neurotypical therapists need awareness that these interests are usually a source of comfort or delight for the autistic individual, and as such they constitute a mental health support. Attwood (2003, p. 126) accurately observed that personal interests "can be perceived as a problem and will then remain a barrier – or as a talent and will then become a bridge."

Many autistic individuals have a lexicon of personal words they have created, or familiar words they use differently than neurotypicals in daily conversation. Attwood (1998, p. 82) noted the ability of autistic children to offer "a novel perspective on language". Such words regularly become integrated into the family vernacular, during childhood, becoming integral to the family culture and thereby contributing to the neurodivergent child's sense of belonging. Neurotypicals encountering such words often recognize them as highly effective descriptors of the item or phenomenon in question. Some examples of these (with gratitude to the neurodivergent individuals who shared them with me) include the following:

- **Twistation** – an uncomfortable knot of bedding that is gradually tightening around the legs or feet, usually at night
- **Insistinel** – a personal imperative
- **Wedgie** – a fold of fabric pressing against the skin, anywhere on the body
- **Thirstacular** – the sensation of extreme thirst
- **Upskin** – eyelid
- **Face meat** – cheek
- **Worm colours** – the opposite of cool colours (because many worm colours are almost the same colour as worms, and because comparing a colour to a temperature just doesn't make sense, according to one – now adult – autistic kid!)

Communication patterns and themes are regularly shared by parents of autistic kids, or neurotypical spouses of autistic adults, within my practice. Parents of autistic kids note with delight and awe the *compelling questions* their young child regularly asks. Existential inquiries such as the exact length of the mail carrier's esophagus, why dead neighbours don't put out their recycling on the appropriate day, and the weight of a brick house, are commonplace.

Another communication-related theme shared by parents and partners is that the *autistic individual rarely requests help.* Since neurotypicals often thrive on feeling needed by the people closest to them, this is a frequent source of relational tension, arising in intimate partnerships as often as in parent-child relationships. Asking for help with challenging tasks is not usually a default behaviour for autistic individuals, which has been explained to me by clients as a combination of a genuine desire to solve the problem oneself, along with an aversion to the idea of having to explain the details of a problem to another person before simply solving it. Consequently, parents of autistic children often describe feelings of confusion when they have observed their child in need of assistance and recognized that asking for help simply did not occur to the child as one potential solution. It is no coincidence that the terms autism and autonomous share the same Latin root.

A third communication theme that regularly arises is that of repeated *scripted communication*, such as snippets of songs or familiar lines from a movie or book. Neurodivergent individuals often enjoy the sounds of certain words or phrases in ways that neurotypicals do not, and experience these sounds as soothing or regulating – additionally so when heard or produced in a predictable rhythm or pattern. Autistic kids have shared in therapy that they "really like the taste" of certain words. Neurotypicals, conversely, often find repetitive sounds boring or irritating, and may have difficulty accommodating their child or partner's need to self-soothe in this way.

In closing this section, a note on *selective mutism* (also known as situational or contextual mutism) is important (Muris & Ollendick, 2021). Selective mutism is an expression of anxiety that manifests as a communication issue, in some autistic individuals. This is an important distinction, because in autistic individuals, selective mutism requires mental health support before (or instead of) speech/language support, as is commonly proposed. Individuals experiencing selective mutism are unable to speak in certain situations or contexts (such as school) but are simultaneously able to speak in more familiar contexts (such as home). Usually present since childhood, the first incidence of selective mutism is often triggered by overwhelming sensory experience or communicative demand at school or elsewhere, and subsequent activation recurs periodically. When it is activated, individuals describe a sensation of profound withdrawal, like a dissociative experience, over which they have no control, and an associated loss of speech. Some individuals can whisper during an episode of situational mutism, but many endorse having no access to speech at all.

During an episode of selective mutism, there is often a strong desire to leave the situation accompanied by a feeling of powerlessness to do so. Many individuals require support from trusted friends or family, to help them leave the situation and create space and time to self-regulate and recover. Written or app-based communication may replace spoken, to reduce the demand for verbal self-expression, and pre-establishing a basic range of gestures with which the individual can convey their needs or safety status, is recommended. Individuals who experience frequent or prolonged periods of selective mutism require NAP to address anxiety, and to increase self-awareness and capacity for self-regulation, alongside their commitment to consistent selfcare. Additionally, their chosen family members or friends may require support and psychoeducation to ensure immediate availability of consistent support, when needed.

Nonverbal communication

Along with verbal communication, non-verbal communication often differs significantly between autistic and allistic (non-autistic) individuals. One of the most widely recognized differences is in social referencing, commonly referred to as "eye contact". Many autistic individuals have significant difficulty with looking directly into another person's eyes, describing the experience on a continuum from uncomfortable to extremely stressful or painful. Trevisan et al. (2017) confirmed that autistic adults and teenagers reported "adverse emotional and physiological reactions, feelings of being invaded, and sensory overload while making eye contact". More confident autistic individuals allow themselves to use an adapted sideways gaze or to avert their gaze fully or intermittently, in social situations where eye contact seems required. However, many others mask by developing compensatory mechanisms such as a fixed gaze, or by directing their gaze at the speaker's nose or chin, to emulate neurotypical eye contact. Unsurprisingly, the ongoing stress thereby experienced by neurodivergent individuals often predisposes them to social anxiety, hypervigilance, or self-deprecating cognitive distortions. The association of direct eye contact with honesty or trustworthiness is a hurtful neuronormative cultural construct that has been intensely damaging to autistic mental health; eye contact is never required of clients in NAP, for any reason.

Trevisan et al. (2017) reported that autistic individuals confirm difficulties with understanding social nuances, as well as difficulties sending and receiving nonverbal information. Autistic individuals, and especially those who identify as female, often develop a range of facial expressions as elements of masking. Many autistic adults recall intentionally developing a "photo-smile" in childhood, to use at family gatherings or picture day at school, when photographs were unavoidable. Photos taken when these individuals were very young often reveal an obvious incongruity between their own facial expression and those of others in the picture, which may have instigated parental disapproval and fueled their decision to develop a fake smile for such moments. Conversely, autistic individuals who mask less frequently (or less intensely) may simply display a narrower range, or more subtle facial expressions, than many neurotypicals. Autistic adults are regularly surprised (or irritated) by neurotypicals asking if they are upset or angry, based upon the neurotypical individual's misinterpretation of their relaxed, focused, or thoughtful facial expression.

Emotional communication

Emotional self-expression is a common area of misunderstanding of autistic communication by neurotypicals, referred to clinically as alexithymia. Individuals with alexithymia endorse great difficulty with feeling, identifying, or expressing emotions, and may have notable difficulty expressing emotions that neurotypicals would consider appropriate to specific social contexts, e.g. sadness or tears at a funeral.[1] Many autistic people describe difficulty with recognizing and expressing their own emotional experience, as well as that of other people, including those closest to them. Often, they report a prolonged delay between the event and their emotional response, resulting in apparent lack of empathy for others' experience and/or lack of support from others when they need it. Some autistic/neurodivergent individuals experience a significant degree of emotional dysregulation, which is also regularly misinterpreted by neurotypicals and subject to discriminatory disciplinary measures in the school years, as well as relational difficulties across the lifespan.

The role of the neurotypical psychotherapist in facilitating communication within a cross-neurotype therapeutic alliance is exactly that: to facilitate communication! As with other cross-cultural communication experiences, the goal is mutual understanding; critically, there can be no agenda to change the neurodivergent client's innate communication style. Neurotypical therapists who bring respect and understanding of autistic communication into the therapy room, provide unconditional acceptance, ample processing time, and demonstrated openness to AAC (Augmentative and Alternative Communication) options such as apps on tablets, laptops and similar, are facilitating cross-neurotype communication in multiple ways. Additionally, those who demonstrate interest and willingness to learn from the client how best to communicate with them, are offering truly accessible psychotherapy. Chapter 9 provides a variety of strategies and techniques that will foster and deepen mutually satisfying communication within a cross-neurotype therapeutic alliance.

Sample therapeutic questions on communication

1. Tell me about a time when you felt heard and understood by someone important to you. (OR, Tell me about a time when you felt like someone else was having difficulty understanding you.)
2. What personal strategies do you use to manage social gatherings like weddings and birthday parties? Do those strategies also work in your professional life, or have you developed others for work-related meetings?
3. When you were a child, what was your favourite story book or movie? Were you allowed to read/listen/watch it as often as you wanted to? Who limited your access to your story/movie, and why?
4. Who was your best friend in elementary school? Do you have any photos of you and your friend that we could look at together?
5. What is communication like between you and your partner? How do you express appreciation for one another? How do you resolve conflict?
6. Are there specific places where you feel more comfortable or relaxed with other people than usual? What makes that place (or people) comfortable company for you? What do you or they intentionally do, to make it so?
7. Do you use any form of AAC? Would it be helpful if we used AAC in session? Would you be willing to show me how to connect with you using AAC,

and help me to recognize moments when you need us to communicate in that way?

7. What is important for me to know about your experience with communication in childhood? In adulthood? In social situations? At work or at school?

Note

1 www.autistica.org.uk/what-is-autism/anxiety-and-autism-hub/alexithymia

References

American Psychiatric Association. (2022). *Diagnostic and statistical manual of mental disorders*. American Psychiatric Association. https://doi.org/10.1176/APPI. BOOKS.9780890425596

Attwood, T. (1998). *Asperger's syndrome: A guide for parents and professionals*. Jessica Kingsley Publications.

Attwood, T. (2003). Understanding and managing circumscribed interests. In M. Prior (Ed.), *Learning and behavior problems in Asperger syndrome* (pp. 126–147). The Guilford Press.

Billeiter, K. B., & Froiland, J. M. (2023). Diversity of intelligence is the norm within the Autism spectrum: Full scale intelligence scores among children with ASD. *Child Psychiatry & Human Development*, 54, 1094–1101.

Bowlby, J. (1979). The Bowlby-Ainsworth attachment theory. *Behavioral and Brain Sciences*, 2(4), 637–638.

De Clercq, H., Jordan, R., Hume, K., & Roberts, J. (2019). Analysis of what makes a successful professional in Autism. In *The SAGE handbook of Autism and education*. Sage Publication Ltd. https://doi.org/10.4135/9781526470409.n8

Doove, B. M., Feron, F. J. M., van Os, J., & Drukker, M. (2021). Preschool communication: Early identification of concerns about Preschool language development and social participation. *Frontiers in Public Health*, 8, 546536. https://doi.org/10.3389/fpubh.2020.546536

Fogel, A. (1993). *Developing through relationships*. University of Chicago Press.

Gutstein, S. (2009). *The RDI book*. The Connections Center.

Gutstein, S. E. (2000). *Autism Aspergers, solving the relationship puzzle: A new developmental program that opens the door to lifelong social & emotional growth*. Future Horizons.

Harrop, C., Amsbary, J., Towner-Wright, S., Reichow, B., & Boyd, B. A. (2019). That's what I like: The use of circumscribed interests within interventions for individuals with autism spectrum disorder. A systematic review. *Research in Autism Spectrum Disorders*, 57, 63–86. https://doi.org/10.1016/J.RASD.2018.09.008

Hartman, L. M., Farahani, M., Moore, A., Manzoor, A., & Hartman, B. L. (2023). Organizational benefits of neurodiversity: Preliminary findings on autism and the bystander effect. *Autism Research*, 16(10), 1989–2001. https://doi.org/10.1002/AUR.3012

Hobson, H., Cross, M., Jefferies, V., & Forster, M. (2022). What is the future of research on language and communication needs and mental health? A report by the Special Interest Research Group for Language, Communication and Mental Health. *Language and Communications SIRG*. (Updated December 12, 2022). In Mental Health Weekly Digest (page 614). https://doi.org/10.31234/OSF.IO/SDF8N

Ilyka, D., Johnson, M. H., & Lloyd-Fox, S. (2021). Infant social interactions and brain development: A systematic review. *Neuroscience and Biobehavioral Reviews, 130*, 448–469.

James, I. (2005). *Asperger's syndrome and high achievement: Some very remarkable people*. Jessica Kingsley Publishers.

Karakaş, N. M., & Dağlı, F. Ş. (2019). The importance of attachment in infant and influencing factors. *Turkish Archives of Pediatrics, 54*(2), 76–81.

Klin, A., Danovitch, J. H., Merz, A. B., & Volkmar, F. R. (2007). Circumscribed interests in higher functioning individuals with autism spectrum disorders: An exploratory study. *Research and Practice for Persons with Severe Disabilities, 32*(2), 89–100. https://doi.org/10.2511/RPSD.32.2.89

Lapakko, D. (2007). Communication is 93% nonverbal: An urban legend proliferates. *Communication and Theater Association of Minnesota Journal, 34*(1), 7–19.

Main, M. (1996). Introduction to the special section on attachment and psychopathology: 2. Overview of the field of attachment. *Journal of Consulting and Clinical Psychology, 64*(2), 237–243. https://doi.org/10.1037/0022-006X.64.2.237

Mehrabian, A. (1972). *Nonverbal communication* (1st ed.). Routledge.

Mehrabian, A., & Ferris, S. R. (1967). Inference of attitudes from nonverbal communication in two channels. *Journal of Consulting Psychology, 31*(3), 248–252.

Muris, P., & Ollendick, T. H. (2021). Selective mutism and its relations to social anxiety disorder and autism spectrum disorder. *Clinical Child and Family Psychology Review, 24*(2), 294–325.

Parsons, C. E., Young, K. S., Murray, L., Stein, A., & Kringelbach, M. L. (2010). The functional neuroanatomy of the evolving parent-infant relationship. *Progress in Neurobiology, 91*, 220–241. https://doi.org/10.1016/j.pneurobio.2010.03.001

Rees, C. (2007). Childhood attachment. *British Journal of General Practice, 57*(544), 920–922.

Trevisan, D. A., Roberts, N., Lin, C., & Birmingham, E. (2017). How do adults and teens with self-declared Autism Spectrum Disorder experience eye contact? A qualitative analysis of first-hand accounts. *PLoS ONE, 12*(11), e0188446. https://doi.org/10.1371/journal.pone.0188446, www.ncbi.nlm.nih.gov/pmc/articles/PMC5705114/

Ulmer-Yaniv, A., Waidergoren, S., Shaked, A., Salomon, R., & Feldman, R. (2022). Neural representation of the parent–child attachment from infancy to adulthood. *Social Cognitive and Affective Neuroscience, 17*(7), 609–624.

Chapter 7

Executive functioning and autistic mental health

Executive functioning challenges are arguably the least apparent and the most disabling features of autism/neurodivergence given the pace and complexity of the dominant culture. With varying ability to organize and manage thoughts, ideas, roles, and personal and shared belongings, and rapid shifting into overwhelm and dysregulation, comes increased vulnerability to debilitating mental health difficulties for autistic/neurodivergent individuals. In this chapter, clinicians are provided with information to increase their understanding of executive functioning, along with guidance on informal assessment of executive functioning issues, informing case conceptualization and treatment planning and delivery. This chapter introduces Attention-Deficit Hyperactivity Disorder (ADHD) as a common comorbidity of autism, a stand-alone neurodiversity, and predominantly, as a disorder of executive functioning.

This chapter responds to the following clinical questions:

1. What does *executive functioning* refer to, and how does it affect mental health?
2. What cognitive/emotional concerns commonly arise for neurodivergent clients when examining their own executive functioning in psychotherapy?
3. Why is Neurodiversity-Affirming Psychotherapy (NAP) a *trauma-informed* approach?
4. How does activation of the *limbic system* impact executive functioning?
5. What happens when executive functioning capacity is exceeded, and what kind of therapeutic support is indicated in NAP?

Introducing executive functioning

Working safely and effectively with autistic/neurodivergent clients requires an understanding of the brain-based concept generally referred to as executive functioning. Suchy described executive functioning as "a multifaceted neuropsychological construct that can be defined as (1) forming, (2) maintaining, and

DOI: 10.4324/9781003430476-7

(3) shifting mental sets, corresponding to the abilities to (1) reason and generate goals and plans, (2) maintain focus and motivation to follow through with goals and plans, and (3) flexibly alter goals and plans in response to changing contingencies" (2009, p. 106). In other words, executive functioning refers to the ability to know what needs to be done, and to just do it! Viewed as such, it is not difficult to recognize the role executive functioning plays in any individual's self-concept, in every life context. Executive functioning refers to the complex arrangement of mental skills and processes required for planning, organizing and prioritizing information; for cognitive shifting; time management; self-monitoring; and dynamically adjusting effort accordingly (Predescu et al., 2020), for following directions, collaboration, goal setting, as well as self-regulation, initiation, and self-inhibition (Diamond, 2013). Clearly, this area of mental functioning has widespread impact on multiple domains, and when it is working well, is associated with feelings of capability and competence for most people. It therefore also has the potential to significantly support, or undermine, mental health. Importantly within NAP, executive functioning is reduced or over-extended to some extent in all neurodivergent individuals, the impacts of which are often reflected in personal disorganisation, challenges with time management and self-deprecating personal narratives, arising in therapy and elsewhere.

In educational parlance, executive functioning is often described as the "manager" of the brain. Hewitson (2018, p. 20) defined it as "the set of mental skills that allow us to problem-solve, plan, organize, switch focus, self-regulate and control our impulses". Paxton & Estay (2007, p. 64) added the mental processes of "self-monitoring and dynamically adapting one's performance or output", to the list. Eaton (2018, p. 118) described executive functioning as "higher-order cognitive abilities such as working memory, planning, flexibility and organizational ability, in terms of both problem-solving and emotional regulation". There is consensus on the vital role of executive functioning then, for individuals to optimize their personal array of cognitive, emotional, and physiological resources, and it is a small step from here to imagine the potential for difficulties when executive functioning is not working optimally, for any individual.

In the context of NAP it is imperative to highlight that commonly held assessments of neurodivergent clients as change-averse or resistant to treatment are usually evidence of executive functioning difficulties, rather than any disrespect for the clinician's time, or a lax attitude to psychotherapy. Neurotypical clinicians need to recognize their clients' individual challenges in this area of mental functioning and use this information to strengthen and protect the therapeutic alliance. Neurodivergent adults often bring a complicated and discouraging history of relational experiences to therapy, much of which reflects executive functioning difficulties that have not been well-understood by the client themselves, nor by important people in their lives. This underscores the importance of the clinician's awareness of this issue, to provide an accessible therapeutic alliance within which the client will have opportunities to challenge their narratives about relationships, and specifically about their own functioning within relationships that matter to them.

Airport analogy for executive functioning

It may be helpful to offer an analogy to demonstrate the role of executive functioning in mental health. This complex set of mental skills and abilities might be compared to an orchestra; every instrument plays a unique part in the music, but a good conductor is essential to ensuring that the result is an uplifting symphony, rather than a mess of discordant chaos! Or, it could be compared to a sports team, where every player has their position, and all are dependent upon the coach for planning, direction, and optimal use of their individual and collective strengths on a dynamic basis. Orchestras and sports teams notwithstanding, this therapist/author is a traveller – and the departure lounge of any international airport provides excellent material for reflection on the importance of executive functioning to mental health. Additionally, it provides vivid examples of what can happen when things are suddenly not operating smoothly enough to meet the level of demand within a complex system.

In the airport analogy, there are two distinct elements: the terminal building and the control tower. The terminal represents an individual's cognitive, physical, spiritual, and emotional functioning – everything they think, feel, and do on an ongoing basis. The control tower represents executive functioning – the director or controller of all such functions! Within this airport, all day and much of the night, there are countless events happening simultaneously, both in the terminal and outside on the tarmac. Many of these events are only apparent to individuals who are directly involved, or hold responsibility for the outcomes, and they generally proceed smoothly and outside the awareness of travellers and most of the airport personnel.

However efficient, attractive, comfortable, or entertaining our imagined airport facility may be, there is consensus that safety is the top priority, taking precedence over all else. For aircraft to land or take off safely, it is imperative that the control tower is fully operational, staffed with well-trained individuals and equipped with updated and well-maintained technology. If the control tower has less than full functionality for any reason, even for short periods, safety is compromised. Everything must come to a halt in the terminal and on the tarmac until the problem is identified and addressed, operations resume, communication is flowing, and safety is re-established. And if a halt is not called, there will be chaos, confusion, and significant danger, within minutes. Although very few people appreciate flight delays, it is reasonable to propose that most would prefer to postpone travelling, to arriving or departing from an airport in the absence of steady, reliable guidance from a well-functioning control tower! Likewise, in the absence of efficient and effective executive functioning, the cognitive, physical, spiritual, and emotional capacity of the individual is compromised, sometimes to the point of complete shutdown. Such is the critical role of executive functioning, and such is its capacity to either support or disrupt mental health and wellbeing.

Executive functioning and neurodivergence

In the absence of known cognitive or physical challenges (e.g. traumatic brain injury, global developmental delay, Down Syndrome, etc.) it is clinically appropriate to hypothesize that when a neurodivergent individual repeatedly feels frustrated or unfulfilled, or believes they are not reaching their potential in significant life tasks (education, career, relationships, etc.), it may be attributable to executive functioning difficulties. For any person, the repeated experience of knowing what one wants (or is expected) to do, but finding oneself struggling to plan, organize, and initiate it, or to follow it through to completion, negatively impacts mental health. Coming into therapy, this is the lived experience for many, arguably most, neurodivergent individuals.

The neurodivergent community online, and elsewhere, shares a wealth of experience on this topic. Many neurodivergent individuals are familiar with the frustration that arises, when they know they have the cognitive resources to solve a problem, create something extraordinary, or contribute original ideas to a collaborative project – but find themselves unable to access those resources under time pressure, or in aversive sensory environments, or when juggling multiple demands, as neurotypicals seem to do with relative ease. Rampant distractibility, difficulties with mental organisation and decision-making, or hyperfocus on specific details or ideas, often stand in the way of assessing the project or task as good-enough, in favour of moving forward. And the neurotypical world generally devalues this level of attention to detail, expansive thinking, and creative processing, obsessed as it tends to be with deadlines, productivity, and efficiency.

In NAP, psychotherapists meet these frustrated, depleted or disenchanted, neurodivergent individuals regularly. They are the quiet, autistic student in grade three, who withdraws from class discussions, finding it pointless to inter-ject with peers whose executive functioning allows them to express an ever-flowing stream of thoughts and ideas ("although they are usually wrong", as one young client has pointed out in session!). They are the autistic adults who converse with depth and insight with one person at a time in quiet settings or outdoors, but avoid work-related, social, and family gatherings because inter-acting with groups disproportionately depletes their personal resources. They are the competent and loving autistic parent who brings home a bouncy puppy with the intention of providing their kids with a beloved pet but find themselves completely overwhelmed and unable to decide whether, who and how to ask for help, and frozen by confusion, indecision, and shame. And they are the autistic professionals who excel in their fields of expertise but cannot manage their time and energy resources efficiently enough to financially support themselves. For autistic/neurodivergent individuals such as these, the obstacles to mental health and life satisfaction are not intelligence, skills, nor ability; they are in prioritizing, planning, organizing and effectively communicating the considerable intelligence, skills, and abilities they clearly have. Their struggle to participate in and contribute to all that matters in their lives without completely depleting their personal resources in the process, calls upon neurodiversity-affirming psychotherapists to recognise, accommodate, and advocate for recognition of the critical role of executive functioning in mental health.

Executive functioning and limbic activation

Returning to the airport analogy, the demands of daily life present all of us with an ongoing stream of cognitive, physical, and emotional challenges, some planned and others unexpected. The internal control tower we refer to as *executive functioning* is responsible for attending, responding, planning, organising, prioritising, and reprioritising dynamically, as the individual navigates the airfield of their own life. At the same time, that control tower must maintain clear, ongoing communication between itself and the rest of the system, ensuring sensory and emotional self-regulation, a sense of competency, resilience to adversity, and access to healthy coping strategies and mechanisms. When the system is working well, the individual enjoys a state of mental health – life is not without problems, but they feel equipped to manage whatever is presented in healthy, adaptive ways. In this healthy state, significant mental activity is ongoing within the *prefrontal cortex* in the area largely dedicated to executive functioning: assessing, thinking, reasoning, decision-making, self-inhibition, and so forth (Yuan & Raz, 2014).

However, when the system stops functioning optimally due to reduced or compromised capacity, prolonged stress or sudden unanticipated overload, the *limbic system* is activated, and temporarily but completely hijacks the control tower! A "state of emergency" is declared; the prefrontal cortex shuts down, and regardless of the individual's overall intelligence or usual resourcefulness, in this state, they will be unable to use their executive functioning to navigate the situation. For excellent reasons to do with the survival of the species, activation of the *limbic system* temporarily deactivates the *prefrontal cortex* (where executive functioning happens). When this happens, multiple physiological changes occur rapidly, as the brain and body prepare for danger; the brain is bathed in cortisol and the body in adrenaline (the so-called "stress hormones"). Along with the temporary shut-down of the "thinking brain", the visual field narrows, blood is diverted to the limbs, body temperature drops, digestion pauses and heart rate increases (Perry & Winfrey, 2021). This cortical shutdown makes sense from a survival perspective, because in moments of great danger, rational thinking and planning are unhelpful – what is required is an instantaneous reaction that readies the body for action, and it is the limbic system that makes this happen. Limbic functioning is straightforward, limiting the individual to just four possible reactions: fight, flight, freeze, or fawn (Pittman & Karle, 2015), but rendering their customary coping mechanisms – observing, thinking, decision-making – temporarily unavailable. This summarises the well-documented "trauma response" (Levine et al., 2018; Perry & Winfrey, 2021) that occurs in all humans when danger is perceived. It is a highly adaptive response to actual danger, but a less-helpful response to perceived or imagined danger, notably, the limbic system cannot distinguish one from the other.

Limbic activation and the associated experience of losing access to one's cognitive abilities is particularly distressing for autistic individuals because of their propensity to rely heavily on their own cognition for their sense of safety and wellbeing. When this domain is suddenly foggy or inaccessible, many autistic individuals demonstrate extreme expressions of anxiety, which may include physical and emotional withdrawal, selective mutism, or panic attacks, any of which may constitute another step toward autistic burnout, the mental health crisis described in Chapter 3. Unlike somatic or emotionally focussed modalities, a strengths-based approach to working with autistic/neurodivergent individuals in psychotherapy centres the cognitive domain as a source of stability and safety, and a springboard for self-understanding and self-acceptance. For autistic clients, having a grasp of reliable information and awareness of how they are processing it is a legitimate pathway toward the aforementioned "state of mental well-being, that enables a person to cope with the stresses of life, realise their abilities, learn and work well, and contribute to their community" (World Health Organization, 2022a).

Resilience and overload

Resilience may be understood as the capacity to manage incremental, excessive, or prolonged stress without limbic activation, and it is a recognized antidote to mental health problems (Zautra et al., 2008). For many reasons, including neurotype, genetic loading, lived experience, effectiveness of self-care, substance use, presence/absence of support systems, and underlying belief systems, individuals have various degrees of resilience from day to day, in different contexts and across the lifespan. And often, neurodivergent individuals experience daily life as somewhat more stressful than neurotypicals, depleting their overall capacity for resilience accordingly.

Most adults have at some point experienced incidents or periods of overload in life; times when their resilience is reduced, or their stress load becomes too great, and a sense of overwhelm pervades. Such periods are inevitable, occurring when a loved-one is very sick, a personal or professional partnership dissolves, an important exam goes awry, or a job or home is lost. They also occur at less apparent moments, when fending off illness or allergens, worrying about current events, navigating school or work-related stress, or struggling within relationships. These challenging times may be compounded by the conviction that one's struggle is invisible to others, perhaps even one's closest supporters, and by the reality that alongside the excessive stress, life's regular set of demands and responsibilities have not magically abated and must still be attended to. For many individuals, feelings of anxiety are common at such times, and may be exacerbated by negativity or isolation. At such times, executive functioning is compromised, causing additional stress for the individual, as an ironic outcome of the original overload of stress. Details are forgotten, keys are lost, forgetfulness or fuzzy thinking sets in. Just as the individual needs the support of clear and efficient executive functioning, it suddenly becomes less available.

Many autistic/neurodivergent individuals experience this kind of overwhelm much sooner than neurotypicals do, because of the multiplicity of external demands that deplete their resources and undermine their resilience, daily. Executive functioning mediates between what a person can do and what they do, in the domains of thinking, memory, attention, and self-regulation – and overload compromises whatever executive functioning resources are usually available to any individual. Because they contribute to an overall sense of competency and efficacy, difficulties in these domains affects mental health. Given the prevalence of executive functioning difficulties in neurodivergent individuals, and the additional stress they experience just navigating life in the dominant culture, this is a critical area for validation, support, and accommodation, in NAP.

Trauma and executive functioning

Trauma-informed frameworks for mental healthcare have radically improved therapy outcomes (Classen & Clark, 2017) for traumatised individuals, families, organisations, and entire systems. The essential elements of trauma-informed care are safety, trustworthiness, choice, collaboration, and empowerment (Butler et al., 2011). NAP is a *trauma-informed approach* to supporting neurodivergent individuals in counselling and psychotherapy.

Trauma, a term that literally refers to a "wound" or "injury", has been extensively researched and its impacts on both the human brain and mind have been demonstrated and validated in recent years. Clinicians and researchers such as Levine et al. (2018), Fisher (2014), Van der Kolk (2003), and Perry (2007) have fundamentally changed the ways psychotherapists understand how the brain is changed by trauma, how those impacts show up in mental and practical functioning, and how to care for the brain and the mind after a traumatic experience.

Trauma is succinctly defined by the American Psychological Association (APA) as "an emotional response to a terrible event like an accident, rape, or natural disaster."[1] However, trauma-informed clinicians recognize that an experience of trauma changes the brain in complex ways, depending on whether it is acute (sudden, unexpected, recent), chronic (in the past, repeated over a period), or complex (occurring in childhood, or involving emotional/developmental damage). The Centre for Addiction and Mental Health (CAMH) offers a more nuanced definition of trauma, which may be more applicable to psychotherapy, as, "the lasting emotional response that often results from living through a distressing event".[2] The important distinction between these two definitions is that the second acknowledges not only the *emotional,* but also the prolonged *temporal element* of the impacts of trauma. Long past the initial traumatic event or experience, emotional responses to comparable experiences or situations can unexpectedly overwhelm the individual, activating the limbic system (fight, flight, freeze, or fawn) and shutting down the prefrontal cortex (executive functioning). One of the important goals of trauma-informed therapy is to raise the client's awareness of such impacts, to support the client in self-compassion, and to equip them with strategies with which to manage trauma responses, when needed. Trauma can be physical, emotional, psychological, or spiritual in nature, and although it is poorly recognized, most neurodivergent clients come to psychotherapy with histories that include experiences of *relational trauma.*

Relational trauma may be understood as mental trauma (or injury) inflicted on a child by their primary caregivers, intentionally or otherwise, literally *by the experience of being in relationship* (Benamer & White, 2018). Relational trauma is common in individuals with lived experience in child protection services, where children have experienced loss or separation from their primary caregivers, often after experiences of abuse or neglect, but are then rehomed and may receive sub-optimal caregiving. Relational trauma occurs when a young child experiences neglect, abuse, or inconsistency of care, from the adults upon whom they are dependent for wellbeing, comfort, and, in infancy, basic survival. Without trauma-informed, relational intervention, the attachment-related outcomes of relational trauma are likely to devastate the child's future relational experiences.

With recognition and gratitude to the many committed and caring foster families that provide excellent care for children, there is ample evidence that kids in care are often moved repeatedly, with little or no opportunity for closure or continuity of important relationships (Ball et al., 2021). Such early life experiences naturally result in insecure attachment patterns and relational behaviour (chaotic/disorganized or anxious/avoidant) (Bowlby, 1979, 1988; Crowell &

Waters, 1994). Individuals whose earliest experiences of being cared-for were frightening or inconsistent will continue to experience caring and being cared-for, as threatening and unsafe (Hughes & Baylin, 2012). Tragically, the mental association of dependency and caring with chaos and instability becomes a relational template for an individual with these experiences, which is perpetuated by a pattern of negative relational behaviours and experiences as they grow up (Hughes & Baylin, 2012; Phillips & Melim, 2020). Extensive support and work in attachment-based psychotherapy provides such individuals opportunities to rewire the trauma-based neural pathways formed in infancy and childhood, allowing them to begin to trust the experience of being consistently cared for, and caring for others, and changing their own relational experience and behaviour accordingly.

A disquieting but comparable experience of relational trauma happens in childhood for many neurodivergent individuals, *even when they are raised by caring parents and within loving families.* It is not uncommon to hear neurodivergent clients in therapy share that their parents dearly loved them but did not fully understand nor accept them. Many bring shame-based personal narratives into therapy, absorbed from spoken and unspoken messages from adults that they were more challenging, complicated, or oppositional than their neurotypical siblings or peers (Pearson et al., 2023). Neurodivergent children have different psychological, environmental, and communication needs than neurotypicals, which may not have been recognised, understood, or met within their family and home. Without neurodiversity-informed guidance or support, it may have taken neurotypical parents many years to recognize that their neurodivergent child's executive functioning needs, intertwined with the sensory and social demands of family life, required a different kind of parenting than they had anticipated. Not uncommonly, parents were aware that something was amiss, but were without the resources to meet the neurodivergent child's needs, and it was expected that the child would adapt to the neuronormative family culture accordingly. In different scenarios, neurodivergent kids with neurodivergent parents may have received negative messages that reflected the parents' own early life challenges, inadvertently (or overtly) promoting masking or camouflaging as approved or necessary coping mechanisms. Whether intentional or otherwise, and whether recognized or not, relational trauma is a common experience in the early lives of neurodivergent individuals, simply as a result of being who they were, and it requires recognition and care, in NAP.

Autistic/neurodivergent children often experience relational difficulties beyond their immediate family. Holliday-Willey (1999) described the behaviour and struggles that result from "pretending to be normal". Referred to as masking or camouflaging (Cook et al., 2021), this complex coping mechanism, utilised consciously or unconsciously by autistic individuals, was explored in Chapter 3. It refers to the individual's propensity to adopt behaviours and mannerisms that they observe in neurotypical peers, with the hope of greater acceptance by those peers (Chapman et al., 2022). Most young children are highly motivated to feel a sense of belonging, and to be included. However, autistic/neurodivergent kids often experience betrayals of trust by peers and adults, and repeated reminders of their social and communication differences from the neurotypical "norm". They are vulnerable to teasing and bullying (Hebron et al., 2015) and are regularly singled out by others as weird or different. As they move through elementary school, they are frequently excluded from social activities and gatherings, and reminded (intentionally or inadvertently) by important adults that they are difficult to parent, to teach, and sometimes, nonsensically but excruciatingly, even to love.

Standard clinical practices are likely to re-traumatise people with trauma histories (Butler et al., 2011), which explains why it is reasonable to assume that every neurodivergent client has a history of trauma coming into therapy, whether they name it as such or not. Many neurodivergent clients have histories of both relational and physical trauma. In pursuit of conformity, physical trauma in the form of restraining, beating, confining, or isolating is inflicted on many neurodivergent children by caregivers or teachers with the goal of teaching (a misnomer from any perspective) social and academic skills. Neurodivergent children are regularly punished by educators and school administrators for attempting to take care of themselves by leaving unbearable sensory environments. They are targeted for physical beatings by bullies, and often unprotected by adults or peers (Cappadocia et al., 2012), disciplined by dysregulated or misinformed parents, and silenced by the educational and healthcare systems that have repeatedly abandoned and failed them (Husk, 2022). For these reasons, it is imperative that psychotherapists working with neurodivergent clients must conceptualise their needs through a *trauma-informed lens* and competently provide *trauma-informed care*. Any other therapeutic stance places the autistic/neurodivergent client at risk of being *re-traumatised* by the therapeutic alliance, adding to their suffering and complicating their journey to mental health.

Autism and executive functioning

It is reasonable to conclude that autistic clients are probably navigating life with some degree of *executive dysfunction,* although the extent and impact of this varies widely. It can be offset by individualised supports and compensations, and autistic/neurodivergent individuals may arrive in therapy with a range of these already in place. Neurodivergent advocates may fairly object to the suggestion that autistic cognitive processing involves dys-anything (Paige Layle,[3] Price [2022]), and indeed the prefix "dys-" suggests a deficit-focused perspective, which is not optimal. However, in discussing how to understand and meet the mental health needs of neurodivergent clients, it would feel negligent to minimize this common feature of neurodivergence. Psychotherapists are cautioned against generalising but are asked to hold this issue in awareness for case conceptualization because its potential for negative mental health impacts in neurodivergent individuals who are immersed in neuronormative cultural milieus, is significant.

An inconclusive body of literature explores the degree to which executive dysfunction is a consistent feature of ASD, present in every diagnosed individual. Demetriou et al. (2018, p. 1198) conducted a meta-analysis of various aspects of executive dysfunction among autistic individuals, eventually proposing a "broad executive dysfunction in ASD that is relatively stable across development". Fernandez-Prieto et al. (2021, p. 2091) highlighted that executive function "has a mediating effect" among emotional self-regulation, sensory processing, and behaviour. My observations suggest that the autistic individual's capacity for self-regulation and sensory processing on any given day facilitates or impedes the ease with which they can access various elements of executive function. In less clinical terms, this simply means that when autistic/neurodivergent individuals are regulated, they have easier access to their own full capacity for thinking, decision-making, and cognitive shifting – whatever it may be for that individual.

Within the therapy room, autistic/neurodivergent individuals regularly share that their executive functioning challenges feel more like reactions to environmental or social demands, than innate features. These individuals generally hold the position that their executive functioning difficulties are familiar to themselves and are not excessively problematic. They note that when they can attend to their own sensory needs and manage the pace and level of demand in their lives, their executive functioning capacity feels comparable to that of their neurotypical colleagues, friends, or family members. Such individuals often report that with the common exception of time management, when they receive appropriate support to understand their own mental health, and some initial progress toward self-regulation is made, their capacity for executive functioning dramatically improves. In the words of autistic advocate Temple Grandin,[4] "I only have autism when I'm around other people – when I'm by myself it doesn't show up at all!"

As noted, *time management* is one element of executive functioning that is frequently raised by (or observed in) autistic/neurodivergent clients. Autistic individuals report reduced awareness of the passage of time, which has often been apparent to themselves and their families since childhood, sometimes causing practical and relational difficulties at home and elsewhere. Most neurodivergent individuals have many personal stories of conflict or confusion with parents, siblings, teachers, peers, employers, or colleagues, that relate to their sense of time; many have difficulty assessing what they or others can achieve in a specific block of time, or how much time they should allocate to a specific task or responsibility. This difficulty with time management can have negative relational and professional implications, and is often positively correlated with anxiety, in autistic/neurodivergent clients. Practical and clinical strategies to support neurodivergent clients who identify time awareness or management as problematic are offered in Chapter 9.

Dysregulation and attachment

The term *dysregulation* refers to limbic activation – the process of losing access to executive functioning when an overload of stress (or fear) has activated the limbic system, as described in the airport analogy above. Neurodivergent clients may describe this as a *meltdown*, or *shutdown* (Phung et al., 2021). Regardless of specific presentation, this degree of dysregulation is a mental health issue, requiring an appropriate response, followed with long-term support. Regrettably, this is not the response that autistic/neurodivergent kids usually receive from either the healthcare or educational systems.

Many autistic adults recall adverse childhood experiences (ACEs) where they became highly stressed or over-stimulated and were inadequately supported. Consequently, their dysregulation progressed to a *meltdown*; a chaotic emotional and physical experience during which they felt terrified and alone, may have mentally detached or dissociated to cope, and of which they have scattered or no conscious memory. Meltdowns are regular occurrences in the lives of many neurodivergent children. They have been inappropriately normalized as aspects of autism that are to be expected (and may even warrant disciplinary measures), particularly in school settings. However, for the neurodivergent child, the mental health impacts of repeated radical departures from regulated functioning on a regular basis, cannot be overstated. The brain is regularly or repeatedly thrown into limbic functioning in response to cumulative and/or unmanageable stress, with significant associated mental, physical, and social impacts (Tyler, 2012). The incremental impact of repeated episodes of extreme dysregulation predisposes neurodivergent individuals to anxiety disorders, depression, body dysmorphia, disordered eating, and bullying, all of which are disproportionately represented in this demographic (Mahjoob et al., 2023). Daily immersion in aversive sensory environments from which the child cannot escape, fuelled by a simmering awareness of social confusion or inadequacy and by increasing executive functioning demands and inadequate supports, many autistic/neurodivergent children experience limbic activation frequently, at school. And when this happens, autistic/neurodivergent students regularly experience punitive, discriminatory, and additionally traumatising reactions from school staff, further undermining their self-concept and mental health.

Neurodivergent adults may express in therapy what they could not articulate in childhood: meltdowns, by this or any other name, are distressing and damaging experiences. The brain perceives that survival is threatened and reacts;

accordingly, there is no access to executive functioning and no ability to draw upon cognition for reassurance or self-regulation. During a meltdown, no meaningful learning can occur (despite well-meaning adults who augment the stress with questions and commands such as: "What exactly is the problem?" "Use your words!" or "Stop this nonsense!"). In a state of complete overwhelm, the child experiencing a meltdown is unable to access, organise, or express thoughts or feelings, and is equally unable to change behaviour on demand. Unsurprisingly, this often results in a terrifying experience of perceived abandonment, regardless of whether they are physically alone or not. Additionally, meltdowns are often followed by painful experiences of isolation, loneliness, and exhaustion, and even of punishment, predisposing the individual to complex feelings of guilt and shame. As the individual matures and more social learning occurs, the outer appearance of a meltdown often shifts from externalised to internalised expressions of dysregulation and overwhelm. In autistic adults, meltdowns may take the form of self-defeating coping mechanisms such as withdrawal from support systems, restrictive eating patterns, substance use, self-harm, or suicidal ideation.

Parents of neurodivergent kids often suffer, regularly observing their child spiralling toward a meltdown, and feeling frustrated with their inability to effectively support the child to self-regulate. Many parents develop a shame-based response to this experience and adapt their parenting to a version of walking on eggshells. Personal boundaries and behavioural limits are inconsistent, which is unhelpful to the autistic/neurodivergent child and everyone else in the family. The mental health ramifications of this family dynamic are extensive. An unsustainable and unhealthy cycle develops: the neurodivergent child's sensory and executive functioning needs are poorly understood and therefore unmet; severe dysregulation occurs frequently, disrupting and limiting family life; a sense of parental inadequacy develops, which is often a precursor to poor mental health in both parent and child (Mahjoob et al., 2023). In extreme cases, a sense of parental inadequacy results in a state of *blocked care* (Hughes & Baylin, 2012) – where the parent is unable to form or sustain a secure attachment relationship with their neurodivergent child. The long-term impacts of insecure attachment in primary relationships is well documented (Bowlby, 1979, 1988; Main, 1996) constituting an added barrier to the formation and sustenance of satisfying adult relationships for the neurodivergent individual.

Attention-Deficit Hyperactivity Disorder (ADHD) and executive functioning

As previously noted, many neurodivergent diagnoses exert such demand on executive functioning as to make it difficult for the individual to find or maintain a sense of inner security and balance, day to day. Autistic/neurodivergent individuals with co-occurring diagnoses such as anxiety, tic disorders (Tourette's Syndrome), depression, substance use disorders (SUD), disordered eating/sleeping, seizure disorders (epilepsy), and/or gastro-intestinal disorders are at higher risk of compromised executive functioning, with associated impacts on mental health. This, in concert with recognition of the many neurodivergent individuals who are undiagnosed but keenly aware of their own processing needs and challenges, spotlights the importance of facilitating neurodivergent clients in recognising, understanding, and managing their individual executive functioning profile and associated needs. Without appropriate support, the mental health of an autistic/neurodivergent individual is likely to eventually be undermined by the strain of managing the executive functioning demands of daily life.

From a psychotherapeutic perspective, it is interesting to wonder whether neurodivergence necessarily compromises executive functioning, or whether the highly sensitive profile (Aron, 2013) of the neurodivergent individual is simply differently focussed; perhaps insightful and aware enough to not waste its resources on managing the ridiculous demands, pace, and complexity of post-modern life. Gabor Maté (2011) spotlighted the impacts of ongoing stress on a system that is simply not designed to manage it – breakdown is inevitable, and the outcomes are likely to devastate both mental and physical health. Irrespective of whether this chicken or its egg comes first, it is clear that the unrelenting stress experienced by autistic/neurodivergent individuals as a result of executive functioning overload constitutes a steady drain on the individual's personal resources, reducing their sense of personal and professional efficacy, heightening anxiety, and undermining mental health accordingly. This drain must be offset by a robust and consistent set of coping strategies, individualised to meet the person's specific needs, and adapted across time to meet the fluctuating demands of their life. Examples of such strategies are offered in Chapter 8, for clinical and personal use, and neurodivergent clients themselves will have personal coping mechanisms, that they may share in therapy. The neurodivergent community online is also an excellent resource for clients seeking support, connection, and resource sharing with peers and allies.

ADHD is of particular significance in discussing executive functioning. A recognised neurodivergent diagnosis, ADHD is also a commonly co-occurring diagnosis among the autistic population. A meta-analysis of the literature by Rong et al. (2021) assessed the prevalence of ADHD in the autistic population at 38.5%, while Hours et al. (2022) proposed that 50 to 70% of autistic individuals are navigating life with co-occurring ADHD. In my own clinical practice, most autistic clients have ADHD, and my observation has been that the two diagnoses together generally place more strain on mental health than either one by itself.

Solden & Frank (2019, p. xi) aptly described ADHD as "dysregulation of the executive function system and related skills". Individuals with the Inattentive subtype struggle with organisation, memory, time management, initiating activity, placing/sustaining attention, and, unsurprisingly, emotional regulation.

Those with the Hyperactive/Impulsive subtype have difficulty staying still, waiting in line, delaying gratification, inhibiting their own actions, or thinking before acting, and often experience a frequent or constant sense of inner restlessness, sometimes described as similar to a low-grade but persistent state of generalised anxiety. Individuals managing the Combined presentation of ADHD experience a blend of features of both the Inattentive and Hyperactive/Impulsive presentations, and the associated challenges.

The impacts of ADHD on executive functioning have implications for every area of cognitive, emotional, and physical functioning. Clients with ADHD may report rapid, incomplete, disorganised, or unhelpful thoughts (cognitive domain), heightened or muted emotional experience and self-expression (emotional domain), and hyper/hypoactive activity and/or discordant communication (behavioural domain). Alongside these difficulties, they may bring significant strengths, unusual abilities, and "outside-the-box" thinking into the therapy room; one of my clients with ADHD has commented that if there is such a box somewhere they certainly have never found it and have neither time nor interest in looking for it! Many ADHD-ers have an unusual capacity for conceptualising and solving problems in unique and original ways. They are most likely to thrive as adults by attending to self-care while centring their own creativity and generativity, instead of continuing to view it through someone else's problem-saturated lens; people with ADHD usually benefit from increasing personal routines in their own lives.

While neurodiversity-affirming therapists will recognise the potential for a relatively short distance between ADHD and poor mental health, it is equally important for them to remember that every journey can be travelled in both directions. For neurotypical therapists working with neurodivergent clients, the challenge lies in facilitating change for an individual whose brain is working differently from their own. Lest it not be obvious, it is unhelpful to suggest that a autistic/neurodivergent client "get organised" or "stop daydreaming"; in fact, such suggestions may constitute microaggressions (Sue, 2010) toward neurodivergent individuals. In particular, when the client has ADHD such comments disregard the client's lived experience, minimise their struggle, and impart a sense of inadequacy and shame in a moment where genuine curiosity, support, and validation are urgently required.

ADHD and medication

ADHD is a significantly disabling condition in terms of executive functioning, but at the client and their physician's discretion, it can be medically treated. Many neurodivergent individuals note that their ADHD is successfully managed with a consistent set of self-care and self-management strategies (learned in psychotherapy or elsewhere) or with a combination of these strategies plus medication prescribed and monitored by their physician. Psychotherapy clients benefit from their therapist's awareness that ADHD medication alone, without lifestyle changes, is unlikely to produce long-term, sustained improvement in mental health.

Psychotherapists do not prescribe medication but require a basic understanding of medications their clients are taking or considering. Much information is available online about medication for ADHD, which generally fall into three categories based on how they work within the brain. These categories are stimulant; non-stimulant; and "other" – the third group being the least commonly prescribed, and sometimes including off-label treatment approaches (see Canadian ADHD Resource Alliance,[5] National Health Service[6]). The presence of multiple neurodivergent features such as tics, migraine or seizure influences or dictates the appropriate medication protocol, so clients are strongly encouraged to share such details with their prescribing physician. Additionally, neurodivergent clients should be encouraged and supported to self-advocate by requesting an extended medical appointment to discuss medication, to bring a written list of their questions to medical appointments, to inquire about the doctor's experience with the needs and sensitivities of neurodivergent individuals, and to request written information/notes about properly using their medication, expected outcomes, and assessing and managing potential side effects.

Non-autistic individuals with ADHD have varying experiences with medication, often trying several different kinds and doses before finding one that works well for them without debilitating side effects. Many autistic individuals have an additionally challenging or frustrating trial-and-error experience with ADHD medication. Not uncommonly, autistic individuals with ADHD and their doctors take some time to find the correct dose of medication for their specific needs, and sometimes a combination of medications is the solution. These highly sensitive individuals may need encouragement and support to ask their doctor to start them on an extremely low dose of ADHD medication, stimulant or otherwise. One of my adult clients describes hers as a "baby dose", having worked extensively with her doctor to find the exact blend and amount of medication, and optimal times of day to take it, that is now enabling her to excel at university while maintaining her mental and physical health, and without unacceptable side effects. Every client using or intending to use medication as part of their ADHD management requires a collaborative, long-term relationship with their prescribing physician, for safety and wellbeing.

Sample therapeutic questions on executive functioning

1. Are you familiar with the concept of executive functioning? (If not, psychoeducation is indicated).
2. Are there areas of your own executive functioning that are more effective than others? Tell me about an area of executive functioning you believe had a positive (or negative) impact on relationships in your life.

3. How often are you on time for important meetings or gatherings? What strategies do you use to monitor time, and how well do they work for you and the people who matter to you?

4. How do you remember important appointments? What did you do to get to this appointment on time today? Is there anything you need me to do to help you to remember our appointments?

5. Who does the planning when you and your partner are going on vacation? How does it feel to you when plans change suddenly? How do you cope with those feelings and that situation?

6. Do you know whether you have ADHD? How does ADHD impact your life and relationships? How do you manage your ADHD, and how well are those strategies working? In what areas do you need a different strategy?

7. Do you take medication for ADHD, and how well does it work? Do you have side effects or other concerns to discuss with your doctor?

8, Would you describe yourself as a resilient person? Please tell me more about your response to this question.

9. What happens when you are extremely stressed or overwhelmed? How will I know if you are becoming stressed in session? What do you need from me or others when you feel overwhelmed?

10. How did people respond when you were overwhelmed as a child? How did you wish they would respond? Who knew what you needed when you felt overwhelmed in childhood?

11. What kind of ADHD do you have (hyperactive/impulsive, inattentive, or combined type), and how does it impact your daily life?

Notes

1 www.apa.org/topics/trauma/
2 www.camh.ca/en/health-info/mental-illness-and-addiction-index/trauma
3 www.paigelayle.ca/
4 Included in a presentation by Grandin, attended by me, in Toronto in 2006.
5 www.caddra.ca/
6 www.nhs.uk/conditions/attention-deficit-hyperactivity-disorder-adhd/treatment/

References

Aron, E. N. (2013). *The highly sensitive person: How to thrive when the world over-whelms you*. Kensington Publishing.

Ball, B., Sevillano, L., Faulkner, M., & Belseth, T. (2021). Agency, genuine support, and emotional connection: Experiences that promote relational permanency in foster care. *Children and Youth Services Review, 121*, 105852.

Benamer, S., & White, K. (2018). *Trauma and attachment*. Routledge.

Bowlby, J. (1979). The Bowlby-Ainsworth attachment theory. *Behavioral and Brain Sciences, 2*(4), 637–638.

Bowlby, J. (1988). *A secure base: Parent-child attachment and healthy human develop-ment*. Basic Books.

Butler, L. D., Critelli, F. M., & Rinfrette, E. S. (2011). Trauma-informed care and mental health. *Directions in Psychiatry, 31*(3), 197–212.

Cappadocia, M. C., Weiss, J. A., & Pepler, D. (2012). Bullying experiences among children and youth with autism spectrum disorders. *Journal of Autism and Developmental Disorders, 42*, 266–277.

Chapman, L., Rose, K., Hull, L., & Mandy, W. (2022). "I want to fit in… but I don't want to change myself fundamentally": A qualitative exploration of the relationship between masking and mental health for autistic teenagers. *Research in Autism Spectrum Disorders, 99,*, 102069.

Classen, C. C., & Clark, C. S. (2017). Trauma-informed care. In S. N. Gold (Ed.), *APA handbook of trauma psychology: Trauma practice* (pp. 515–541). American Psychological Association.

Cook, J., Hull, L., Crane, L., & Mandy, W. (2021). Camouflaging in autism: A systematic review. *Clinical Psychology Review, 89,*, 102080.

Crowell, J. A., & Waters, E. (1994). Bowlby's theory grown up: The role of attachment in adult love relationships. *Psychological Inquiry, 5*(1), 31–34. https://doi.org/10.1207/S15327965PLI0501_4

Demetriou, E. A., Lampit, A., Quintana, D. S., Naismith, S. L., Song, Y. J. C., Pye, J. E., Hickie, I., & Guastella, A. J. (2018). Autism spectrum disorders: A meta-analysis of executive function. *Molecular Psychiatry, 23*(5), 1198–1204. https://doi.org/10.1038/mp.2017.75

Diamond, A. (2013). Executive functions. *Annual Review of Psychology, 64*, 135–168. https://doi.org/10.1146/ANNUREV-PSYCH-113011-143750

Eaton, J. (2018). *A guide to mental health issues in girls and young women on the autism spectrum: Diagnosis, intervention, and family support*. Jessica Kingsley.

Fernandez-Prieto, M., Moreira, C., Cruz, S., Campos, V., Martínez-Regueiro, R., Taboada, M., Carracedo, A., & Sampaio, A. (2021). Executive functioning: A mediator between sensory processing and behaviour in Autism spectrum disorder. *Journal of Autism and Developmental Disorders, 51*(6), 2091–2103. https://doi.org/10.1007/S10803-020-04648-4

Fisher, J. (2014). Putting the pieces together: 25 years of learning trauma treatment. *Psychotherapy Networker, 38*(3), 33–39.

Hebron, J., Humphrey, N., & Oldfield, J. (2015). Vulnerability to bullying of children with autism spectrum conditions in mainstream education: A multi-informant qualitative exploration. *Journal of Research in Special Educational Needs, 15*(3), 185–193.

Hewitson, J. (2018). *Autism: How to raise a happy autistic child*. Orion Spring.

Holliday-Willey, L. (1999). Pretending to be normal: Living with Asperger's Syndrome. Jessica Kingsley Pub, UK.

Hours, C., Recasens, C., & Baleyte, J.-M. (2022). ASD and ADHD comorbidity: What are we talking about? *Frontiers in Psychiatry, 13*. https://doi.org/10.3389/FPSYT.2022.837424

Hughes, D. A., & Baylin, J. (2012). *Brain-based parenting: The neuroscience of caregiving for healthy attachment*. WW Norton & Company.

Husk, S. A. (2022). Cutting the IDEA's Gordian Knot: Accepting entanglements of disability and self and embracing a" best interests" approach to disciplining students with disabilities. *Journal of Law and Education, 51*, 86–143.

Levine, P. A., Blakeslee, A., & Sylvae, J. (2018). Reintegrating fragmentation of the primitive self: Discussion of "Somatic experiencing." *Psychoanalytic Dialogues, 28*(5), 620–628.

Mahjoob, M., Paul, T., Carbone, J., Bokadia, H., Cardy, R. E., Kassam, S., Anagnostou, E., Andrade, B. F., Penner, M., & Kushki, A. (2023). Predictors of health-related quality of life in neurodivergent children: A systematic review. *Clinical Child and Family Psychology Review, 27*(1), 91–129. https://doi.org/10.1007/S10567-023-00462-3

Main, M. (1996). Introduction to the special section on attachment and psychopathology: 2. Overview of the field of attachment. *Journal of Consulting and Clinical Psychology, 64*(2), 237–243. https://doi.org/10.1037/0022-006X.64.2.237

Maté, G. (2011). *When the body says no: The cost of hidden stress*. Vintage Canada.

Paxton, K., & Estay, I. A. (2007). *Counselling people on the autism spectrum: A practical manual*. Jessica Kingsley.

Pearson, A., Rose, K., & Rees, J. (2023). 'I felt like I deserved it because I was autistic': Understanding the impact of interpersonal victimisation in the lives of autistic people. *Autism, 27*(2), 500–511.

Perry, B. D. (2007). Stress, trauma and post-traumatic stress disorders in children. *The Child Trauma Academy, 17*, 42–57.

Perry, B. D., & Winfrey, O. (2021). *What Happened to You?: Conversations on Trauma, Resilience, and Healing*. Flatiron Books: An Oprah Book.

Phillips, S., & Melim, D. (2020). *Belonging: A relationship-based approach for trauma-informed education*. Rowman & Littlefield Publishers.

Phung, J., Penner, M., Pirlot, C., & Welch, C. (2021). What I wish you knew: Insights on burnout, inertia, meltdown, and shutdown from autistic youth. *Frontiers in Psychology, 12*, 741421.

Pittman, C. M., & Karle, E. M. (2015). *Rewiring the anxious brain. How to use the neuroscience of fear to end anxiety, panic and worry*. New Harbinger Publications.

Predescu, E., Sipos, R., Costescu, C. A., Ciocan, A., & Rus, D. I. (2020). Executive functions and emotion regulation in attention-deficit/hyperactivity disorder and borderline intellectual disability. *Journal of Clinical Medicine, 9*(4), 986. https://doi.org/10.3390/JCM9040986

Price. D. (2022). *Unmasking autism: Discovering the new faces of neurodiversity*. Harmony.

Rong, Y., Yang, C. J., Jin, Y., & Wang, Y. (2021). Prevalence of attention-deficit/hyperactivity disorder in individuals with autism spectrum disorder: A meta-analysis. *Research in Autism Spectrum Disorders, 83*(3), 101759. https://doi.org/10.1016/J.RASD.2021.101759

Solden, S., & Frank, M. (2019). *A radical guide for women with ADHD: Embrace neurodiversity, live boldly and break through barriers*. New Harbinger.

Suchy, Y. (2009). Executive functioning: Overview, assessment, and research issues for non-neuropsychologists. *Annals of Behavioral Medicine: A Publication of the Society of Behavioral Medicine, 37*(2), 106–116. https://doi.org/10.1007/S12160-009-9097-4

Sue, D. W. (2010). *Microaggressions and marginality: Manifestation, dynamics, and impact* (D. W. Sue, Ed.). John Wiley & Sons.

Tyler, T. A. (2012). The limbic model of systemic trauma. *Journal of Social Work Practice*, *26*(1), 125–138.

Van der Kolk, B. A. (2003). *Psychological trauma*. American Psychiatric Pub.

World Health Organization. (2022a). *Mental Health Fact Sheet*. United Nations.

Yuan, P., & Raz, N. (2014). Prefrontal cortex and executive functions in healthy adults: A meta-analysis of structural neuroimaging studies. *Neuroscience & Biobehavioral Reviews*, *42*, 180–192.

Zautra, A. J., Hall, J. S., Murray, K. E., & Resilience Solutions Group 1. (2008). Resilience: A new integrative approach to health and mental health research. *Health Psychology Review*, *2*(1), 41–64.

Therapeutic tools of Neurodiversity-Affirming Psychotherapy (NAP)

Every detail is significant, when aligning a therapeutic practice with NAP principles. Colours on office walls ... placement of furniture ... ambiance of the waiting area ... proximity of a kitchen within the building ... construction in the neighbourhood... tone of voice and structure of initial questions ... these and an array of other issues and environmental characteristics can have profound influence upon the cross-neurotype therapeutic alliance, and upon the success of the autistic/neurodivergent client's path toward improved mental health in our care. This chapter provides practical guidance on specific strategies and techniques that align with NAP and can be implemented in any clinical setting; advises clinicians on assessing their usual clinical practices for accessibility to autistic/ neurodivergent individuals; invites reflective practice on connecting these adaptations with the sensory, communication, and executive functioning aspects of neurodivergence, and informs advocacy within the context of the dominant neuronormative culture. Multiple experience- and evidence-based strategies and protocols are provided that will guide clinicians, and students, in adapting their clinical practice and preparatory study for NAP. The chapter closes with a point-form summary of the salient aspects of NAP for easy reference.

Chapter 8 responds to the following clinical questions:

1. How is understanding *sensory processing* among neurodivergent individuals integrated into NAP?
2. What *practical strategies* may be undertaken by the therapist to prepare the therapeutic environment for NAP?
3. How is *effective communication* endorsed and adapted in NAP?
4. How is *executive functioning* supported among neurodivergent individuals in NAP?
5. In sum, what are the *distinctive, pivotal elements* of the NAP approach?

Psychotherapy is a relational endeavour; there is no one-size-fits-all approach, and the common factors paradigm (Wampold, 2015) enables and requires each

DOI: 10.4324/9781003430476-8

client/therapist partnership to undertake a unique and individualized journey together. Psychotherapy is also a cultural endeavour; the bond between client and therapist, an essential element of the therapeutic alliance, is strengthened by the therapist's capacity and willingness to explore and challenge the assumptions of the dominant culture.

Every client brings a unique set of concerns, life events and the meanings assigned to them, access to support systems, and varying needs and goals into the therapy room. Clients come to psychotherapy seeking help to make change, often to increase contentment or decrease suffering, in their own lives. The common factors for change in psychotherapy are the bond between therapist and client, the goals articulated by the client, and the pathway proposed by the therapist (Wampold, 2015) on which they will travel towards those goals. It is incumbent upon the therapist to have an idea of the terrain on the pathway they propose, and of common obstacles and areas of ease, along the way. While theoretical soundness along with the therapist's own experience with their proposed path may render it somewhat familiar, every client brings a particular set of challenges making the journey interesting, challenging and ultimately rewarding, for both travellers. Additionally, every therapeutic pathway will occasionally be splashed with droplets from a rambunctious little creek that flows alongside, calling the therapist's attention to the distinct needs of the individual client, in psychotherapy. In NAP, those droplets call upon the therapist to reflect upon their role and capacity to provide neurodivergent clients with opportunities to increase their self-awareness and capacity for self-regulation, within the process of working towards their known therapeutic goals. *In NAP, working toward the client's goals while supporting increased self-awareness and facility with self-regulation are interconnected processes, integral to the model.*

Awareness and understanding of the sensory, communication, and executive functioning elements of neurodiversity leads many clinicians naturally to a critical and creative exploration of their own work, their clinical environment, what happens for autistic/neurodivergent individuals within it, and how such individuals have typically/previously responded to this experience. If a team or setting is fortunate to include some neurodivergent clinicians, or even a neurotypical with neurodivergent family members, these individuals are likely to support an organizational shift toward neurodiversity-affirming practice; indubitably, it will benefit everybody.

Endorsing sensory processing within NAP

When adapting a clinical setting to provide NAP, the *sensory environment* is a good starting point, for three reasons. Firstly, an intolerable sensory experience can put an untimely (or immediate) end to therapy for a highly sensitive individual. Secondly, therapists as well as clients benefit from working in a sensory-friendly environment. And lastly, the sensory environment is the quickest and easiest element of NAP for therapists and clinic administrators to attend to, requiring little more than a basic awareness of sensory processing, some good intentions, and a very small budget. Recognizing that every individual's sensory profile is unique, and that what is helpful to one person will be less or more helpful to another, it is reasonable to propose that the following sensory-based adaptations to any clinical space will improve accessibility for most autistic/neurodivergent individuals, while remaining largely unnoticed or ignored by most neurotypicals.

The visual sense (sight)

Many neurodivergent individuals have visual hypersensitivity; autistic individuals regularly endorse bright or flashing lights and geometric visual patterns as sources of fatigue, stress, and even pain. Conversely, some neurodivergent individuals seek visual input by watching ceiling fans, toys with flashing lights, or screen-based games. Many neurodivergent individuals express uncertainty around their visual hypersensitivity. Parmar et al. (2021) demonstrated that autistic adults who understand their own visual processing needs experience less anxiety about them than those who don't, highlighting the importance of therapist awareness and psychoeducation when working with neurodivergent individuals in therapy. Practical strategies to accommodate visual hypersensitivity include:

- Minimize movement and activity in shared spaces, especially the waiting area.
- Ensure floor coverings and furniture are plain or minimally patterned (avoiding strong, geometric patterns) and ideally made from natural materials.
- Replace horizontal blinds with curtains or solid-coloured window coverings.
- Reduce lighting: if it is necessary to augment natural light, use incandescent bulbs with dimmer switches. Remove fluorescent bulbs and strip-lighting.
- Position furniture so clients are not directly facing a light source; position yourself so you are not back-lit, even with natural light.
- If the client comes in wearing sunglasses, or with a peaked cap, recognise these as necessary for self-care of visual hypersensitivity.
- Cover striped radiators with plain material such as wood or fabric.
- Avoid reflective surfaces, such as large mirrors and ceramic tiles, etc.
- Sit in the same place for sessions and maintain a consistent backdrop/surrounding.
- Position yourself so clients can unobtrusively avert their gaze in session.

- Avoid rearranging furniture between sessions (if furniture must be moved, tell the client before entering that the room looks different; allow extra time at the start of the session for the client to visually reorientate to the space).
- Supply paper and pens/pencils. Invite and encourage autistic/neurodivergent clients to record anything they want to remember, and to make lists of things they plan to do.
- Welcome clients to support their own attention and engagement by doodling or drawing during sessions; provide the necessary materials.
- Encourage clients to try journaling (in words, pictures, or video) to continue processing their therapeutic work between sessions.
- Use signage to convey perpetual requests: e.g. *Please remove wet footwear here.*
- Support executive functioning by writing the client an e-mail or narrative letter (Epston, 1994) after particularly important or impactful sessions.

The auditory sense (hearing)

Many neurodivergent individuals have great difficulty filtering out extraneous sound. Managing competing auditory stimuli in the environment helps neurodivergent clients place/maintain their attention on the therapeutic process.

- Reduce or eliminate unnecessary sound in the therapy room, waiting area, and hallways: prioritize fixing dripping taps, squeaking fans, rattling chairs and toilets that run continuously after they have been flushed! Remove ticking clocks, bubbling fish tanks or indoor fountains Avoid streamed entertainment and require headphones for personal devices in the waiting area.
- Dampen extraneous sound with foam sound excluders below doors.
- Avoid "white-noise machines" if possible.
- Advocate with colleagues who are unaware of their own noisy habits.
- Limit eating and drinking to non-public areas.

The tactile sense (touch)

Many autistic/neurodivergent individuals find soft textures soothing, and often have a somewhat limited selection of preferred clothing. For example, they may own multiple identical t-shirts or sweaters to increase their physical comfort during their day.

- Provide soft comfort objects, including stuffed toys and cushions of all sizes.
- Position both a fleece blanket and a weighted blanket within the client's reach.
- Have multiple fidget items with varying textures within easy reach (reach for one yourself, occasionally!).

- Have a clean bedsheet or towel available to cover furniture for clients who find the texture of upholstery aversive.
- If the client arrives wearing a fitted hat, cap or other head covering, welcome this as self-care for tactile hypersensitivity.
- If you use a desk or floor fan in hot weather, set it to a non-oscillating mode.
- With client agreement, the presence of a cat, dog, or any (quiet) animal is welcome in NAP.

The gustatory sense (taste)

Specific, familiar tastes can be comforting for many neurodivergent individuals and may encourage a relaxed state in the therapeutic environment.

- Offer cold water or a warm beverage to self-regulate in session.
- Welcome the client to snack, chew gum or suck candy, to self-regulate in session.

The olfactory sense (smell)

Many odours that are unobtrusive (or pleasant) for neurotypical individuals are offensive to neurodivergent people and may constitute a significant barrier to NAP.

- Ask the client if there are specific smells they find aversive; assure them you will endeavour to ensure they are not subjected to those smells during therapy.
- Avoid scented personal care products: shampoo, lotion, perfume, deodorant, etc.
- Close windows if food or other environmental smells can be detected.
- Refrain from using scented candles, air fresheners and cleaning products.
- Ask the client if there are specific smells they enjoy/find comforting; explore ways to incorporate those scents into the therapeutic experience.
- Install new furniture and carpets with windows open for off-gassing.
- Post signage requesting accommodation of sensory sensitivities in shared spaces.

The proprioceptive and vestibular systems (body position, effort, balance)

Many neurodivergent individuals benefit from physical movement, deep pressure, balance, or resistance activities before and during mental activity. Physical activity is an important pathway to self-regulation and enhanced engagement and is often unavailable (or considered unacceptable) in workplaces/classrooms.

Explore ways to welcome self-care in the form of physical activity. Provide a selection of equipment to enable clients to explore the self-regulatory effects of different kinds of proprioceptive input.

- Provide and incorporate a springboard, trampoline, weighted blanket, exercise ball and bands, medicine ball, wobble board, beanbag, or ball chair, rocking chair, yoga mat, etc.
- Demonstrate comfort with movement: standing, stretching, changing seat, etc.
- Welcome clients to sit on the floor if they prefer it to a chair, and join them!
- Place a coffee table or similar between client and therapist to support clients for whom assessing/establishing personal space is challenging.

The interoceptive system (information about the body or mind, from within the body)

Opportunities to develop or improve interoceptive awareness may arise organically in NAP, particularly when clients have difficulty feeling/locating emotions in their bodies. Neurodivergent clients who identify increased self-awareness as a goal of therapy may benefit from quietly listening to their own breathing, tracking their pulse, or monitoring digestive sounds and feelings, in the context of therapy. NAP is enhanced by having the following items available:

- A stethoscope and/or magnifying glass.
- A music source, with space to dance or stretch, and a yoga mat.
- Mindfulness-based activities on individual cards or recordings.
- Pre-printed body outlines for locating/mapping emotion in body.

Additionally, see Chapter 5 on highlighting the role of sensory processing in mental health among autistic/neurodivergent individuals.

Endorsing communication within NAP

Communication is the second area to which some initial, broad brushstrokes are appropriate, in preparing to provide NAP. Communication is in the bedrock of the therapeutic alliance; each therapist and client partnership will find or create a common language to facilitate engagement and monitor progress toward the client's desired change. As highlighted in Chapter 3, emergence of the therapeutic alliance requires a bond between therapist and client, along with clarity on the goals of therapy and the tasks by which those goals will be met (Imel & Wampold, 2008). With respect to the client-therapist bond, Cravener (1992) appropriately emphasized that, especially when therapist and client have different cultural backgrounds, establishing rapport depends on the clinician's ability to communicate empathic understanding of the client's feelings and belief systems. At the same time, any therapist's ability to communicate empathy is only as effective as their client's ability to receive and process that communication as intended. Pinto et al. (2012) demonstrated that client-centred interaction styles enhance the therapeutic alliance by facilitating the client's reception of emotional support. Clearly, if our intention is for clients to understand and reflect on whatever we are communicating, we need to communicate it in their own language. *In NAP, therapists communicate in ways that are accessible and meaningful to autistic/neurodivergent individuals.*

It is apposite to reiterate that the purpose of NAP is to lay the foundation for a robust therapeutic alliance between a client and therapist with different neurotypes, within which they can work together to facilitate the changes the client wants to make, in their own life. It is essential that neurotypical therapists recognize, reflect, and regularly remind themselves that at no time are we "treating" autism, nor any other diagnosis, in NAP. When a client and therapist have different neurotypes, communication is an obvious potential stumbling block; NAP is appropriately positioned as cross-cultural psychotherapy. As such, the onus is on the neurotypical therapist as a member of the dominant culture, to learn how to communicate with the neurodivergent client in ways that create safety, space, and ease within the therapeutic alliance.

There is no specific vocabulary therapists are required to adopt in NAP; however, there are unquestionably communication styles that can either impede, or facilitate, the work. An appropriate style of communication is developed through heightened awareness and avoidance of cultural aspects of communication that exclude autistic/neurodivergent individuals. It also requires self-awareness, and willingness to intentionally adjust one's own communication, when necessary.

Collins & Arthur (2017, p. 29) remind therapists that "the enactment of social justice entails relinquishing the privileging of our own perspectives, a rigorous and sometimes painful self-examination". Neurotypical therapists are invited to take up this opportunity for growth, by capturing and reflecting on moments when communication falters between them and an autistic/neurodivergent client. Communication breakdown is a common and uncomfortable experience for neurodivergent individuals within the dominant neurotypical culture. Many autistic individuals have difficulty accessing neurotypical forms of communication repair (e.g. acknowledging momentary distraction or requesting that a question be repeated or rephrased), and often benefit from exploring ways they may do this without shame, in therapy. Within the therapeutic alliance, the uncertainty that communication breakdown generates in therapist or client is potentially a harbinger of insight for both parties, when openly identified and respectfully explored. Learning to tolerate such uncertainty and to investigate it with curiosity is fertile ground for growth, self-compassion, and reduction of shame. *In NAP, therapists develop or increase their competency in cross-cultural communication, in service of deepening the therapeutic alliance.*

Adapting communication for NAP

The following methods and considerations will be helpful in preparing for and conducting effective communication in NAP.

- Self-regulate before and throughout sessions with autistic/neurodivergent clients.
- Articulate the norms or rules of your practice within the Client Agreement and set aside time to clarify the client's understanding.
- Speak slightly more slowly than you usually speak and pause more often. Monitor the client's level of engagement and adapt as needed to ensure you stay together.
- Recognize that neurodivergent clients may interpret facial expressions and communicative gestures differently than neurotypicals.
- Recognize that neurodivergent clients may experience tone of voice and volume differently than neurotypicals.
- Welcome and intentionally create short periods of silence within sessions.
- Know that clients with ADHD may interrupt, complete, or answer a question before you finish asking it. Recognize this as a brain-based difficulty with self-inhibition.
- Know that autistic clients may benefit from prolonged processing time (5–10 seconds) before responding, especially to a direct question. Recognize this as hyperfocus.
- Remain quiet after asking a question; refrain from repeating or rephrasing it unless the client asks you to do so.
- Write down (or invite the client to write down) anything they want to remember; do not rely on auditory memory exclusively, for important information.
- Use direct communication: ask or say specifically what you mean (see examples below).

The following paragraphs provide examples of adaptations to neurotypical communication that may strengthen the therapeutic alliance with neurodivergent clients. In each example, the therapist is intentional about supporting the client's memory, while communicating their question or comment briefly, clearly, and specifically. Intentionally decluttering verbal communication usually reduces anxiety and facilitates self-regulation in neurodivergent individuals. Consider the following:

Instead of: I've worked hard to provide an environment that is responsive to the needs of people with sensory sensitivities, so I hope you will give me some feedback on anything that is helpful or not; please tell me if there's anything you need to feel comfortable in this space.

Say: Look around and help yourself to anything you need to feel comfortable.

Instead of: How are you doing today? What is on your mind today?
    Ask: What is *on your list* of things to discuss today?

Instead of: How did you feel after our last session? Did you have more thoughts later?
    Try: Last time, we talked a lot *about fishing.* Did you have more thoughts *about fishing* since then?

Instead of: I wonder if she started to get a bit confused with all those details…
    Offer: That topic is important to you. *What did she do or say to show you that she understood?*

See Chapter 6 for therapeutic questions that develop/enhance a neurodiversity-affirming communication style.

Endorsing executive functioning within NAP

Chapter 7 explored the executive functioning features of autism/neurodivergence. It is not difficult to extrapolate the potential impacts of executive functioning difficulties on the neurodivergent individual's education, employment, and relational experience, all of which may undermine mental health and wellbeing. *In NAP, therapists recognize and accommodate executive functioning issues to provide a therapeutic experience that is accessible and helpful to autistic/neurodivergent clients.*

Autistic/neurodivergent individuals whose personal narratives suggest they are (or believe they are) underachieving or underemployed may need specific and ongoing executive functioning support in psychotherapy and beyond, to reach their potential. This is an accessibility requirement for this demographic and is effectively addressed through an individualized blend of psychoeducation, emotional and practical support, and advocacy. Autistic/neurodivergent individuals are often strong self-advocates; however, clients who require support to ask for what they need, within psychotherapy and beyond, are well-supported by a therapist who will walk this piece of the journey with them when needed.

Self-advocacy by young students is usually actively discouraged within school systems. Many autistic/neurodivergent kids have great difficulty navigating educational systems that neither understand nor properly accommodate their executive functioning needs, and school often becomes a prolonged experience of shame and conflict, for them and their families. The social and sensory demands of school are extensive, homework often causes family stress, and the incremental complexity of the curriculum creates steadily increasing difficulties with organization and participation, reducing many autistic/neurodivergent students' opportunity to keep pace with their peers, and to succeed. School history and experiences with self-advocacy are often rich areas for personal exploration, in NAP.

Sometimes, well-intentioned parents or caregivers inadvertently overcompensate for an autistic/neurodivergent child's executive functioning difficulties, organizing every aspect of their life while advocating effectively on their behalf, to the extent that they do not develop their own self-advocacy capacity. Neurodivergence is somewhat heritable, and parents are often highly motivated to protect kids from negative experiences such as they or a sibling had, in their own school years. While completely understandable, a common outcome of parental overcompensation is that it conceals the full extent of the student's executive functioning difficulties, which become starkly apparent when they first attempt to live independently or attend college/university. Some neurodivergent individuals will then experience a period of intense self-doubt, scrambling to manage the multiple challenges and demands of "adulting". Many feel overwhelmed by the organizational aspects of meal planning, shopping, and food preparation. Others struggle to meet deadlines, manage money, make/keep appointments, or remember to do laundry before they have nothing clean to wear. If they are able and willing to receive support, NAP allows these young adults to understand their experience in terms of their executive functioning and helps them explore a variety of strategies to support themselves while adapting to the sudden increased demands of adult life. As they explore self-understanding and self-acceptance, the neurodiversity-affirming psychotherapist supports the individual as needed, in learning to self-advocate in specific situations or at the systemic level, to ensure they have equal access to the opportunities and choices that are available to their neurotypical peers. For some young adults, taking a break from school for selfcare and for the autistic/neurodivergent individual and their support people to put structure and routines in place is often an excellent strategy. *In NAP, therapists promote client mental health by participating in systemic and individual advocacy with (or on behalf of) neurodivergent clients.*

Tools of the executive functioning trade

The following practical strategies to support executive functioning have been helpful to many of my clients. Some were introduced to me by autistic/neurodivergent clients, and to those individuals I am grateful; your strategy of choice has helped more people than we will ever know! Other strategies emerged organically while a client and I struggled to tackle a specific executive functioning issue together. With typical neurodivergent processing, several of these strategies gelled long after a session ended, with positive outcomes of collaborative and creative thinking, a little extra processing time, and a wee touch of risk-taking!

An important note: before suggesting strategies to support executive functioning, always explore with the client what strategies they have previously used and whether/how much they helped. Many autistic/neurodivergent individuals have unique and effective ways to support their own self-regulation and executive functioning and may not have identified them as such. Clients may draw or doodle, listen to loud music, work on a jigsaw puzzle, walk in nature, soak in a hot shower or bath, spend time with a beloved pet or sit down and make a Big List. Examine and assess together how well the client's current strategies and personal supports are working, and if it ain't broken, don't fix it! *In NAP, the client's personal support strategies and adaptations are welcomed and sustained.*

The following strategies are used overtly by therapists in NAP and can be suggested/taught to clients who express interest, with the intention that they become resources used in the client's daily life. Many psychotherapists draw from a variety of theoretical backgrounds, enriching their work and positioning them to meet a wide variety of mental health needs. NAP is a transtheoretical model, and as such, elements of multiple evidence-based therapies belong comfortably within it, often without any adaptation required. Clinicians who provide evidence-based attachment therapies such as Emotion-Focused Therapy (EFT) or Internal Family Systems Therapy (IFS) will be on familiar ground here. Additionally, some of the tools and approaches that are commonly used in Narrative Therapy, Acceptance and Commitment Therapy (ACT) and Dialectical Behaviour Therapy (DBT) are helpful to autistic/neurodivergent individuals with minimal adaptation. Harm reduction in NAP involves developing an understanding of the sensory, communication and executive functioning aspects of neurodiversity and filtering case conceptualization and treatment planning through this information. Like all robust therapeutic approaches, it involves clear communication with clients, goal setting and monitoring, intentional self-care, regular clinical supervision, ethical decision-making, measured risk-taking, curiosity, humility, and a genuine desire to help people feel better about themselves and their lives.

Many therapists would agree that a unique blend of existential and practical concerns enter the space with every new client. The remainder of this chapter suggests multiple small but significant techniques therapists can introduce or use to convey acceptance and understanding to autistic/neurodivergent clients, without speaking a word. Aside from supporting executive functioning, these strategies can quietly validate the limbic system's concerns and send it back to bed, calming the chaos and allowing the client's prefrontal cortex to resume effective management of the airport, in everybody's best interests!

Transitioning into therapy

For clients, moving from the waiting area to the therapy room is a *transition,* and autistic/neurodivergent individuals experience different degrees of ease with transitioning. In autistic individuals, this is often attributed to their capacity for *hyperfocus,* which has been described as the "perpetual and unrelenting state of intense single-minded concentration fixated on one thing at a time, to the exclusion of everything else" (Rowland, 2020, p. 2). Autistic adults note there are both advantages and disadvantages to their ability to place their full attention on one topic or activity for prolonged periods, largely depending on the social context (Russell et al., 2019). An autistic/neurodivergent client in a busy waiting area may be immersed in a book or device, requiring a few additional moments to transition from waiting-room mode into walking mode without becoming dysregulated. When a person's natural processing style engages their full attention in whatever they are thinking about, they are often in a state of hyperfocus; they may need more time than others to extract and redirect their attention. This happens each time the individual transitions from work to home, from classroom to recess, and at the start and end of every appointment: autistic/neurodivergent individuals need an extra moment to intentionally shift their attention on demand. *In NAP, clients are invited into appointments quietly, clearly, and without comment when they need 5–10 seconds to stop what they are doing and join the therapist.*

Pausing at the door of the therapy room, the therapist invites the client to look around and share if they see or hear anything that may distract them or cause sensory discomfort. This allows the client to transition more slowly into the space, to assess it through their own sensory experience, and to modify the environment if needed, to reduce sensory disturbance. *In NAP, clients are encouraged to centre their sensory experience, to attend to their sensory needs, and to self-advocate when necessary, on this or any other aspect of therapy.*

The client explores the space visually or physically and decides where they will sit and how they will make themselves comfortable in the space, using the sensory supports the therapist has provided. *In NAP, clients are supported to discover what blends of movement, pressure, texture, temperature, light, sound and even taste, are optimal for self-regulation.* For clients who are regularly deprived of sensory supports in daily life, this discovery may be a therapeutic goal; for others it constitutes an important area of self-care that facilitates cognitive processing, increases self-awareness, and deepens the therapeutic alliance.

The therapist, meanwhile, briefly assesses their own self-regulation and attends to it as needed, to ensure they are fully present and have ample capacity for co-regulation. They also observe how the client has arranged themselves and the things around them, and if a pattern emerges across repeated sessions it is noted. Many autistic clients self-regulate using ritual; a stop at the water cooler, a familiar pair of slippers, or the same cushion to hold on their lap, at every session. These repeating patterns emerge organically and are usually uncomplicated; they are encouraged and valued as key aspects of selfcare, and elements of deepening the therapeutic alliance. *In NAP, therapists facilitate small rituals as elements of a therapeutic experience that has enough predictability to make it accessible to the individual client.*

Routines and habits

Repetition can be an effective support for executive functioning, especially when used to remember and complete boring but necessary areas of functioning such as feeding pets or oneself, doing laundry, taking medication, or personal hygiene. Autistic/neurodivergent individuals often have a natural affinity for patterns and comfort with repetition, and this can be used to their advantage by establishing simple, repetitive habits for things they want (or need) to do or remember. This serves the dual purpose of remembering to do the thing, whatever it may be, and freeing up executive functioning resources for more rewarding or interesting pursuits!

Activities that happen regularly and frequently are more likely to become habitual, and to be remembered. It is worth emphasizing this in NAP because adult clients commonly resist it. Such resistance may be mental clutter from childhood, when habit-forming was insisted upon by adults and became negatively associated with authority figures with unclear or personally meaningless intentions. It is worth investigating and challenging such beliefs with adult clients; simple habits and routines can save time, money, and energy (while preserving preserve one's health or significant relationships in the process!). *In NAP, personally meaningful habits and routines such as sitting in the same place at each appointment are welcomed as positive memory supports.*

Visual and auditory supports

Neurodivergent individuals are often strong visual learners, as evidenced by their overrepresentation in university faculties of engineering, architecture, and design (Wei et al., 2012). Visual strengths can be an asset to therapy, if properly employed. Frequently, clients engage deeply in session, only to leave the room and forget what they experienced, what was discussed or decided, and when they are to return. Due to executive functioning issues, poor short-term (working) memory is a commonly occurring issue in autistic/neurodivergent individuals, often precipitating shame-based responses, and frustration with self and others. Autistic/neurodivergent individuals may have significant difficulty in this area, causing personal distress and relational dissatisfaction, and limiting education and career advancement. This is an important point, because poor short-term memory can also undermine the therapeutic alliance if not recognised, validated, and addressed.

Therapists can provide short-term memory support by intentionally ending sessions a few minutes early to write a short note or reminder of session highlights, which the client can add to a notebook or therapy journal. Writing the note may later become the client's responsibility, with the therapist protecting the necessary time and providing materials. An enriched option to an end-of-session note that provides excellent memory support for neurodivergent clients is a therapeutic letter, such as those written to clients by narrative therapists. Epston (1994) affirmed that "what is made concrete in the session itself is made doubly concrete in the letter".[1] Narrative letters are written by therapists and sent to clients after a session, providing a memory support for the client, and a structured opportunity for the therapist to reflect on the session and draw out the salient threads. Writing narrative letters is a specialized skill, requiring training and supervision; however, a short note highlighting what the therapist observed about the client's progress, and anything they believe the client may want to remember, is an acceptable strategy for any therapist.

The use of visual memory and organizational supports such as lists, charts, diaries/organizers, schedules, and calendars is modelled and encouraged in NAP, as are auditory supports such as voice-activated apps and handheld voice recorders. These low-tech options are safe, inexpensive and accessible, and often effective in reducing anxiety. *In NAP, therapists openly use their own visual memory supports, explore with clients what supports have been effective for them, and encourage discussion and experimentation with a variety of tools.*

A plethora of online apps augment and support executive functioning, many of which are specifically designed for (and by) neurodivergent individuals. Used appropriately, these can reduce overwhelm, and with it the frequency and intensity of dysregulation. Like everything in the online world, the list of available apps increases regularly; some of the current favourites in my practice include Goblin Tools, To-do-ist, Evernote, Trello, and Tick Tick. Neurodivergent clients have identified these as uncluttered, easy to use, and even somewhat adaptive to the user's individual needs. However, a cautionary word to therapists is appropriate here. Neurodivergent individuals may struggle with the challenging aspects of hyperfocus and/or distractibility, and the online world is designed to keep visitors engaged, consuming … and online! Many neurodivergent minds are quickly drawn to the next "shiny object", making it difficult to self-monitor online, and assessment of risk is the therapist's responsibility when suggesting or recommending strategies. Fundamentally, if a therapist has clinical reasons to suspect that any strategy or device may generate additional difficulties for a specific client, suggesting that the client explore it would be unethical clinical practice; careful, individualized consideration is indicated.

Medication reminders

Many individuals with ADHD use a blend of medication and lifestyle adaptations to support executive functioning and reduce overwhelm. Medication for ADHD must be taken at regular intervals to work optimally and minimize side effects; ironically, remembering to take it can be challenging when navigating life with the executive functioning elements of ADHD.

An effective memory support for many neurodivergent individuals using prescription medication is a low-tech device called a *dosette*; a small box which is divided into sections for each day and time, that they take meds. These are available from pharmacies and are routinely filled by the client once a week, or similar. A higher level of support is available for individuals who have difficulty remembering to fill their dosette weekly; on request, pharmacies can dispense medications in "blister packs", pre-labelled with the day and time each dose should be taken. As well as helping clients remember to take their medication, these supports enable them to check retroactively whether they took it, if the appointed day or time has passed and memory does not serve. *In NAP, clients who use medication are supported to do so effectively and safely.*

Cell phones and distractibility

Executive functioning is regularly hijacked by distractibility among clients with ADHD, often manifesting as repeatedly checking their phone for messages, or "doom-scrolling" ostensibly to dampen anxiety. Depending on the degree of distractibility and the impact on the therapeutic alliance (and possibly other relationships), it may be helpful to explore ways to help the client to place and sustain their attention on the process, for the duration of the session. Recognizing that it may be counter-cultural, if electronic devices undermine the bond between client and therapist, it is clinically appropriate for both to intentionally place their electronic communication devices out of sight and hearing during therapy. It is rarely adequate to turn off notifications, and although it may initially cause uncertainty, many autistic/neurodivergent individuals need their device to be invisible, inaudible, and out of reach, to minimize distractions in therapy. It is a worthwhile experiment for an interested client, at minimum!

When engaged in virtual therapy, it is exceedingly difficult for clients with ADHD to resist the notifications that inevitably pop up on their screens. Once the therapeutic alliance is established, this may be an important area for exploration; the client is entitled to know the impact of their sudden (or repeated) departures on the alliance. For some clients this feedback will be unimportant, while for others it will resonate as a familiar source of relational stress that they may decide to address, by using the on/off button or "airplane mode" to full advantage when interacting with significant people in their own lives. *In NAP, the impact of brain-based distractibility on relationships is acknowledged and explored.*

Time management

Since a disproportionate amount of the autistic/neurodivergent individual's energy is required for self-regulation and executive functioning, progress in therapy should be anticipated to take longer than with neurotypical clients.

Additional time is required for cognitive processing, for self-regulation, and for transitions, and the overall pace of therapy cannot exceed the client's capacity to remain engaged with it while navigating competing demands for their attention. Neurodivergent individuals often endorse the relational issues that arise when different neurotypes experience the passage of time, and the allocation of time-related resources, quite differently. Many have experienced relational breakdown that neurotypical partners have attributed to their persistent lateness. Others have learned to compensate by arriving for appointments or meetings unnecessarily early. Both patterns of behaviour are aspects of executive functioning and both can have benefits and drawbacks that can be explored in NAP.

Neurodivergent clients whose capacity for time management is truly debilitating may require additional support from the therapist or clinic to remember, or to arrive on time, for therapy appointments. It is important for therapists to recognize that without additional information, autistic/neurodivergent clients who have difficulty arriving on time for appointments cannot be presumed to be uninvested in therapy. It is much more likely that lateness has been a long-term problem for the individual, has had extensive relational impacts, and originates in a brain-based difficulty with monitoring and managing time; it should be broached accordingly.

As mentioned, psychotherapy with neurodivergent clients is unlikely to progress at the same pace as neurotypicals, whose attentional resources are generally available without much more than a timely cup of coffee to self-regulate. Neurodivergent clients experience discrimination by Employee Assistance Programs (EAPs) and insurers, who often provide just enough coverage for them to become acquainted with a therapist and end their coverage after a mandated six or eight sessions. For neurodivergent individuals to truly benefit from psychotherapy, many require approximately twice as many sessions as neurotypical clients. This allows time for a cross-neurotype therapeutic alliance to emerge and deepen, and for therapy to proceed at a pace and in ways that do not overwhelm the neurodivergent individual's executive functioning capacity. Some autistic/neurodivergent individuals need sessions to be shortened somewhat, and therapy to occur in smaller chunks; others need sessions lengthened, to allow for additional processing and reflection time. *In NAP, awareness and management of time is recognized as an accessibility requirement which is accommodated on an individual basis.*

Decision-making

Decision-making is often a complicated and emotional process for autistic/neurodivergent individuals, and additionally for those with ADHD. If this is an issue for a client, it will become evident in therapy whether they articulate it or not; distress will be apparent when a decision is required. Asked to decide on a practical question (e.g. dates for future sessions) such a client's executive functioning resources will be quickly overloaded by a rapid and extensive flood of possibilities surging forward simultaneously, making the decision impossible and triggering a limbic response in some individuals. Difficulty with decision-making has relational implications, particularly if it is not recognized as an element of neurodivergence, and neurodivergent clients may express confusion or frustration around the apparent ease with which neurotypicals make decisions. *In NAP, clients are supported to investigate their own experience with decision-making, and to experiment with self-regulating while making low-demand decisions within the therapy room.*

Distinctive elements of NAP

The following are highlights of key elements and protocols of NAP, which are described in detail in this chapter:

1. *Working toward the client's goals while supporting increased self-awareness and facility with self-regulation are interconnected processes, integral to the model.*
2. *With client agreement, the presence of a cat, dog, or any quiet animal is welcome in therapy.*
3. *Clients are invited into appointments quietly, clearly, and without comment if they need extra time to shift their attention and join the therapist.*
4. *Clients are encouraged to centre their sensory experience, to attend to their sensory needs, and to self-advocate, when necessary, on this and any other aspect of therapy.*
5. *Clients are invited and supported to discover in therapy what blend of movement, pressure, texture, temperature, light, sound, and even taste, is optimal for their own self-regulation.*
6. *Therapists facilitate small rituals as elements of a therapeutic experience that has enough predictability to make it accessible to the autistic/neurodivergent client.*
7. *Therapists intentionally communicate in ways that are accessible to autistic/neurodivergent individuals.*
8. *Therapists develop competency in cross-neurotype communication in service of deepening the therapeutic alliance.*
9. *Therapists recognize and accommodate executive functioning issues to provide a therapeutic experience that is accessible to autistic/neurodivergent clients.*
10. *Therapists promote client mental health by participating in systemic and individual advocacy with (or on behalf of) neurodivergent clients.*
11. *The client's personal support strategies and adaptations are welcomed and sustained.*

12. *Personally meaningful habits and routines are welcomed as positive ways to support memory.*
13. *Therapists openly use their own visual memory supports, explore with clients about what supports have been effective for them, and encourage discussion and experimentation with a variety of tools for memory support.*
14. *Clients who use medication are supported to do so effectively and safely.*
15. *Impacts of brain-based distractibility on relationships is acknowledged and explored.*
16. *Awareness and management of time is recognized as an accessibility requirement and is accommodated accordingly.*
17. *Clients are supported to investigate their own experience with decision-making, and to self-regulate while making low-demand decisions during therapy.*

This chapter presented practical strategies for providing NAP with autistic/neurodivergent clients. Particular emphases were placed on preparing the therapeutic environment to accommodate autistic/neurodivergent individuals' sensory processing needs; on empathic and culturally appropriate, cross-neurotype communication; and on recognition and accommodation of executive functioning needs. The key distinctive characteristics of NAP were summarized for easy reference by clinicians and students.

Note

1 https://reauthoringteaching.com/about/what-is-narrative-therapy/david-epston-letter-writing/

References

Collins, S., & Arthur, N. (2017). Challenging conversations: Deepening personal and professional commitment to culture-infused and socially just counselling practices. In C. Audet & D. Paré (Eds.), *Social justice and counseling: Discourse in practice* (1st ed.). Routledge.

Cravener, P. (1992). Establishing therapeutic alliance across cultural barriers. *Journal of Psychosocial Nursing and Mental Health Services, 30*(12), 10–14. https://doi.org/10.3928/0279-3695-19921201-05

Epston, D. (1994). Extending the conversation. *Family Therapy Networker Nov/Dec.*

Imel, Z. E., & Wampold, B. E. (2008). The importance of treatment and the science of common factors in psychotherapy. In S. D. Brown & R. W. Lent (Eds.), *Handbook of counseling psychology* (4th ed., pp. 249–266). John Wiley & Sons.

Parmar, K. R., Porter, C. S., Dickinson, C. M., Pelham, J., Baimbridge, P., & Gowen, E. (2021). Visual sensory experiences from the viewpoint of autistic adults. *Frontiers in Psychology, 12,,* 633037. https://doi.org/10.3389/fpsyg.2021.633037

Pinto, R. Z., Ferreira, M. L., Oliveira, V. C., Franco, M. R., Adams, R., Maher, C. G., & Ferreira, P. H. (2012). Patient-centred communication is associated with positive therapeutic alliance: A systematic review. *Journal of Physiotherapy, 58*(2), 77–87. https://doi.org/10.1016/S1836-9553(12)70087-5

Rowland, D. (2020). Redefining autism. *Journal of Neurology, Psychiatry and Brain Research (JNPBR), 02*, 148. https://doi.org/10.37722/JNPABR.20202

Russell, G., Kapp, S. K., Elliott, D., Elphick, C., Gwernan-Jones, R., & Owens, C. (2019). Mapping the autistic advantage from the accounts of adults diagnosed with autism: A qualitative study. *Autism in Adulthood, 1*(2), 124. https://doi.org/10.1089/AUT.2018.0035

Wampold, B. E. (2015). How important are the common factors in psychotherapy? An update. *World Psychiatry, 14*(3), 270. https://doi.org/10.1002/WPS.20238

Wei, X., Yu, J. W., Shattuck, P., McCracken, N., & Blackorby, J. (2012). Science, technology, engineering, and mathematics (STEM) participation among college students with an autism spectrum disorder. *Journal of Autism and Developmental Disorders, 43*(7), 1539–1546. https://doi.org/10.1007/s10803-012-1700-z

Chapter 9

Goal setting and monitoring in Neurodiversity-Affirming Psychotherapy (NAP)

When setting out on a journey, for safety, success, and shared enjoyment, we need to know something about the terrain we will navigate, our means of transport, and benchmarks to notice (and pitfalls to plan for) along the route. When robust mental health is the destination, the therapeutic goals and tasks are the map, and the means of transport is the therapeutic alliance. In cross-neurotype alliances, the most significant potential pitfalls are the gaps of cultural understanding within, and the impact of neuronormativity on, the cross-neurotype alliance. In NAP, almost any obstacle can be navigated, if the therapist is aware of and planning for, these invisible, challenging and eminently navigable potholes!

This chapter provides responses to the following clinical questions:

1. What is the particular importance of *collaborative goal setting* and *progress monitoring* to positive outcomes in NAP?
2. What is the difference between *avoidance goals* and *approach goals*, and why does this matter, in NAP?
3. What constitutes a *SMART goal*, and why is it a useful framework for goal setting in NAP?
4. How does a *strengths-based perspective* of autism/neurodivergence influence goal setting and progress monitoring in NAP?
4. What obstacles are commonly encountered to *collaborative, cross-neurotype goal setting/progress monitoring*? How can neurotypical therapists manage such obstacles in neurodiversity-affirming ways?

The role of goals in therapy

The therapeutic alliance that forms between two individuals (one of whom seeks change, while the other facilitates it) is central to every discussion about what works in psychotherapy. Originally described by Bordin (1979), and extensively revisited and reiterated in the literature since, the therapeutic alliance comprises three elements: (a) the bond between client and therapist; their agreement on

DOI: 10.4324/9781003430476-9

(b) the goals of therapy; and (c) the tasks by which those goals will be pursued. The therapeutic alliance may be conceptualized as a container, easily recognizable to both the client and therapist as a space that is consistently safe, for the shared journey of psychotherapy. This chapter focusses on the importance of therapeutic goals to the alliance and the outcomes of therapy, and on goal setting and monitoring within the cross-neurotype therapeutic alliance.

Setting goals for therapy is an important element of treatment planning with every client (Cooper & Dryden, 2015, p. 35). In NAP, identifying and articulating clear goals, and monitoring progress toward them, respects the autistic/ neurodivergent individual's affinity for clarity, direction, and sufficient predictability, while supporting the neurotypical therapist to stay on track (or to consistently return to the track, when inevitable forays down side trails or off-roading adventures occur!). Mutually acceptable and clearly stated therapeutic goals, and agreement on how progress will be monitored, foster a sense of hope and positive expectancy in clients of all neurotypes. In my experience, many autistic/neurodivergent clients value the experience of collaboratively monitoring their own movement toward their goals; many have reflected in therapy that it provides quantifiable evidence of their personal growth and capacity to choose and capably manage change in their own lives. Importantly, therefore, goal setting and progress monitoring in NAP must happen in ways that are experienced by the autistic/neurodivergent client as empowering and encouraging, rather than obscure or shame-inducing. In psychotherapy, as in life, careful, respectful use of language really matters.

It is reasonable to propose that in general, people feel and cope better when they perceive an element of coherence to the direction of their lives. Positive psychology highlights having (rather than necessarily attaining) goals as one of the conditions for humans to thrive. Conoley and Scheel noted that "growth and flourishing occur under known conditions: involvement in meaningful activities; experiencing supportive, caring relationships; feeling competent; having goals; and experiencing positive emotions frequently" (2017, p. viii). Importantly, however, goals must be personally meaningful to the client, rather than imposed by others. The ways in which client goals are explored and formulated in psychotherapy have an impact on both the client's experience of working with them, and their likelihood of meeting them.

An aspiration, dream or wish is not a goal, although they may be the raw material from which an excellent set of goals will emerge. Goals have specific features that make them useful in facilitating desired change, which will be outlined later in this chapter. Often, the language used by therapists and clients during the goal setting process has a significant impact on the outcomes of therapy. For example, the subtle effect of using language to describe a desire for increased happiness differs significantly from language that describes a desire to decrease anxiety, overwhelm, or confusion, in one's life – although initially the desired outcome may seem identical. Gable (2006) described *avoidance goals* as those that emphasize ceasing to have a problem by finding ways to avoid or escape its painful outcome. Their opposite, referred to as *approach goals*, place emphasis on articulating the goal in terms of what will be increased, added, or attained. Conoley and Scheel (2017, p. 4) highlighted that avoidance goals inevitably keep the client entangled with their problem while struggling to solve it, while approach goals provide the client with an alternative, and desirable, end state. Gable (2006) demonstrated that approach goals are reliably associated with less loneliness and more satisfaction with social connections, whereas avoidance goals are associated with more loneliness, negative social attitudes, and increased relationship insecurity. For these reasons, unless the autistic/neurodivergent client emphatically insists otherwise, NAP formulates client goals in terms of what the client will increase or achieve, rather than what they will reduce or eliminate, with the intention of setting out on a pathway that is likely to optimize client wellbeing while diminishing their psychological distress (Conoley & Scheel, 2017, p. vii). In reality, this or something resembling it, is probably what the client was seeking when they initially requested psychotherapy.

Collaborative goal setting

Collaborative determination of goals and tasks is a core element of Bordin's (1979) formulation of the working alliance. A shared journey that proceeds without a mutually agreed-upon destination is decidedly less likely to lead the travellers to a good place than one that starts out with a destination that appeals to both, and a map to guide the way. Likewise, collaborative goal setting and agreement on the tasks by which those goals will be met, are critical elements of a successful therapeutic journey. Early in the process, clients often find it helpful to explore with their therapist what they believe, imagine, or remember an improvement in their mental health would look or feel like, and to collaborate on setting goals accordingly. Collaborative goal-setting allows therapist and client to orient themselves and their work toward an end-point, or several end-points (which may change along the way). Whether or not the initial goals guide the process from start to finish, aiming toward mental health as the client envisions or defines it, and setting agreed-upon goals that are aligned with that definition or picture, is an ethically sound, client-centred starting place for psychotherapy. And, in cross-neurotype therapy, several unique challenges and opportunities require a little extra consideration, in advance.

Collaboration requires that individuals find ways they can work well together, which often represents an area of difficulty in social and personal life for autistic/ neurodivergent individuals. In the worst-case scenario, attempting to collaborate on goal setting too soon may undermine the nascent bond between a client and therapist with different neurotypes, by triggering intolerable feelings or painful memories in the client, which may be misinterpreted or mishandled by the therapist. Since collaboration cannot happen in the absence of co-regulation, goal setting in NAP is deferred until co-regulation is established, which may first require a period of repeated, low-demand, mutually enjoyable interactions. For this reason, collaborative goal setting often begins later in NAP than in models of therapy where clients and therapist have the same neurotype and therefore tend to co-regulate more quickly and easily.

Plainly put, providing NAP to autistic/neurodivergent individuals requires that the psychotherapist (and the conversation) moves slowly, quietly, and gently at first; we are intentionally prioritizing the formation of the bond with the client over the other two aspects of the therapeutic alliance (goals and tasks). Recognizing that their different neurotypes magnify the inevitable power imbalance between every client and therapist, these adaptations are intended to compensate for the differences in how their individual and different minds are taking in, processing, and responding to their shared experience, moment by moment. Therapists providing NAP attend carefully to the emotional and behavioural cues of autistic/neurodivergent clients, responding in trauma-informed ways to any shift toward dysregulation. Trauma-informed responses including a gentle voice, clear communication of boundaries, calming presence, noticing and care of physical discomfort, welcoming (and modelling) of self-soothing behaviours and provision of a sensory-supportive environment, facilitate co-regulation. Additionally, conveying the lack of demand or time pressure to an autistic/neurodivergent client reduces pressure, often with positive effects on self-regulation and executive functioning. Conversely, moving into collaborative undertakings without first establishing a co-regulated framework is unlikely to result in developing a common language or finding a therapeutic way of being together.

This highlights the reason why collaborative goal setting must be undertaken differently in a cross-neurotype therapeutic alliance, in service of establishing a client-therapist bond that will withstand the journey and enable the client to meet their goals. Hodgetts et al. (2018) noted that although it is well-established that self-determination is linked to social inclusion and improved quality of life for autistic adolescents, those same adolescents were rarely active participants in the goal-setting process in their own therapy. Rather, goal-setting was typically undertaken by their parents and therapists, often generating goals that differed significantly from those the adolescent would have set for themselves. Individuals who have had previously inadequate opportunities for self-determination will require additional space and time in NAP to initially engage with the concept of setting personally meaningful goals and collaboratively creating a plan to pursue them.

Importantly, autistic individuals who received ABA in childhood regularly demonstrate prompt dependency in the therapeutic alliance, as in other important relationships in their lives. Without the therapists' keen and dynamic awareness, in cross-neurotype therapy the potential for perpetuation of prior unhelpful relational patterns is significant, reducing the autistic client's opportunity to engage effectively with psychotherapy. Camilleri et al. (2024) interviewed a group of autistic adults with self-set therapeutic goals. Along with reporting positive outcomes, the participants in this study reported an increased sense of personal agency within their therapeutic experience, which they attributed to being supported to reflect upon, and then to set, their own therapeutic goals. NAP therapists are responsible for ensuring they provide accessible opportunities to autistic clients to collaborate in setting and pursuing goals that are personally meaningful, and genuinely desirable, to them.

Autistic strengths and challenges in collaborative goal setting

As explored in Chapter 2, in tandem with their individual personal assets, experience, and abilities, autistic/neurodivergent individuals have specific strengths that are common to the neurotype and are strong assets to goal setting in NAP and beyond. These often include an affinity for patterns, attention to detail, creative approaches to problem-solving, capacity for deep and sustained attention, systems-based thinking, and often a roguish and impressive sense of humour! By centering and utilizing these assets in the goal-setting process, therapists and clients can generate goals that will serve the client in making the changes they want, in their own life, while safeguarding and strengthening the therapeutic alliance at the same time.

Alongside the strengths that autistic/neurodivergent clients may bring, it is important to also hold in awareness some of the challenging features of neurodivergence in preparing for goal setting. The unusually prolonged early phase of NAP, while co-regulation is explored and established, provides ample opportunity to observe, and explore with the client, the extent to which the communication, sensory processing, and executive functioning elements of neurodivergence may be affecting their personal wellbeing. At the same time, the therapist may reflect on the impacts of these features on the process of collaborative goal setting and plan accordingly.

Sensory processing needs are often identified and addressed in the process of establishing co-regulation, and the sensory environment of the therapy room is adapted accordingly. The **communication** features of autism/neurodivergence show up in the therapy room just as they do in daily life, and holding space for autistic individuals to express themselves with comfort and ease is key to the cross-neurotype therapeutic alliance. For many autistic individuals, unsatisfactory cross-neurotype communication has been significantly painful in important contexts and relationships, causing negative relational experiences and contributing to negative self-concept, unwanted isolation, and loneliness, among other issues. From the outset, NAP intentionally provides the autistic/neurodivergent client with a distinctly different relational experience, which is immediately apparent in the therapist's neurodiversity-affirming communication style, described in detail in Chapter 8. It is always a beautiful moment when it occurs to an autistic/neurodivergent client that there are two people involved in every verbal exchange, each of whom hold about 50% of the responsibility for the direction, comfort, and outcomes of the flow – and no more! Many have anxiously interacted with their own lives carrying a mistaken belief that frequent communication breakdowns between them and others were always "their fault", fueling a negative self-perception that was seeded and repeatedly reinforced by people and systems drenched in neuronormativity. Autistic/neurodivergent individuals who have previously struggled with verbal (expressive and receptive) language, regularly comment on the ease with which they are able to communicate in NAP, inviting a fresh perspective on what they may have experienced in previous interactions, and inviting reflection on how they want to show up in future cross-neurotype exchanges.

The **executive functioning** elements of neurodivergence can add interest to collaborative goal setting, while generating material that may support increased self-awareness/self-understanding, in the client. Goal setting draws on executive functioning, and autistic/neurodivergent individuals who have difficulty organizing their thoughts, prioritizing their concerns, monitoring time, and so forth, may require practical assistance, accommodations and/or additional support in psychotherapy. Such individuals often have a range of shame-based accounts that demonstrate how this aspect of cognitive functioning has impacted their self-concept, and equally, have sometimes developed a creative set of personalized coping strategies. All such strategies that can be incorporated into the goal setting process should be welcomed, except for any that result (intentionally or otherwise) in the therapist taking over the client's share of the work!

It is my experience that many autistic/neurodivergent clients experience a distinct improvement in their overall mental health when supported to recognize their own experience of sensory processing, communication, and executive functioning with curiosity, without judgement, and primarily as aspects of neurodivergence. The shared process of co-regulation followed by collaborative goal setting often provides therapeutic benefit. For many, the impact of neuronormativity has been to cast their neurological profile as inherently problematic, rather than to position it simply as evidence of neurodiversity, across the species. The goals these individuals generate for therapy often become their personal pathways to recasting the model, or reframing the picture, of who they truly are – and intend to be – in the world.

Articulating goals

The range of outcomes that clients desire or anticipate from therapy is essentially limitless. However, the Bern Inventory of Therapeutic Goals (Grosse & Grawe, 2002) suggests that clients' therapeutic goals can generally be categorized into the following five categories:

1. Coping with specific problems and symptoms
2. Interpersonal goals
3. Wellbeing and functioning goals
4. Existential issues
5. Personal growth

In my experience, these categories are similar across neurotypes. What often differs considerably are the beliefs and experiences that autistic/neurodivergent clients hold around goal setting as a general concept. Many neurodivergent individuals initially resist goal setting, which may reflect their difficulty with imagining what life would be like without the problem, because the problem has (or feels as if it has) always been there. Frequent use of the terms "always" and "never" may reflect time-related aspects of executive functioning; as noted previously, neurodivergent individuals often struggle with the time-bound expectations of neuronormativity. As an aside, I have observed that the popularly-used Miracle Question, as employed in Solution Focused Brief Therapy (SFBT, see De Shazer et al., 2021), is rarely helpful to neurodivergent individuals. My hypothesis is that many have difficulty imagining their life without the problem, essentially because the problem is rooted in omnipresent neuronormativity, and not in themselves at all. Additionally, as reflected in Kayrouz and Hansen (2020), more than one autistic individual has responded to this question with a quizzical expression and a very logical statement: "I actually don't believe in miracles".

Occasionally, autistic/neurodivergent clients arrive in therapy with a clear and achievable goal, or several, in mind. More commonly, new clients will have a general goal of "feeling better" or "feeling less anxious". Client and therapist collaborate on clarifying what the client is experiencing, and what they would like to be experiencing, and together will formulate a goal, or several, accordingly. Many neurodivergent clients have difficulty articulating goals for therapy and may have similar difficulty articulating goals in their own lives. It is appropriate and helpful to explore with such individuals the role that setting or pursuing goals has previously played in their lives. Commonly, autistic individuals have had goals imposed upon them by parents/caregiver, the school system, behavioural therapists, healthcare providers, and others, and consequently may find the concept of goal setting off-putting to begin with. Others may experience the therapist's suggestion of a discussion about setting therapeutic goals as a demand they cannot meet, finding themselves suddenly feeling "stuck" in a limbic reaction. Cooper and Dryden (2015, p. 35) suggested that therapist and client simply recognize and accept "stuckness", potentially exploring the idea that simply articulating a goal of any kind may be an appropriate first goal for them, in therapy. When working with autistic/neurodivergent clients, moments of apparent "stuckness" require time, space and careful monitoring, with recognition that the client may need a little more processing time, along with the possibility that they are navigating a highly-anxious response, such as an episode of selective (situational) mutism. In NAP, the arrival of "stuckness" indicates the immediate need to pause, to convey unconditional acceptance, and offer gentle, co-regulatory opportunities, ample time, and encouragement of client self-care.

Integrating strengths and navigating obstacles

A significant majority of autistic individuals are highly observant and strong visual learners. Grandin describes her thought process as "completely visual" (Grandin & Scariano, 1986, p. 131), and Holliday-Willey (1999, p. 48–49) described her use of visual cues to navigate around her university campus. For autistic/neurodivergent individuals who use their visual sense as an asset, the use of a flipchart to organize ideas, and recording of goals on index cards or similar, may be helpful memory and processing supports (white boards should be avoided, as many neurodivergent individuals find the odours of dry-erase markers and cleaning fluids intolerable).

The affinity for patterns that many autistic/neurodivergent individuals report often makes a formulaic approach such as Specific, Measurable, Attainable, Realistic, Time-bound (SMART, see Bovend'Eerdt et al., 2009), an attractive way to articulate goals. SMART goals are used widely in psychotherapy, and in education and business, as a structured way to identify a clear and functional direction for the work. As previously noted, approach goals are more favourable; NAP therapists may suggest re-wording a goal that is proposed by the client to emphasize a positive rather than negative intention. Since many autistic/neurodivergent individuals are detail-oriented, the client is more likely to consider and accept a re-wording if the therapist pays attention to preserving the exact original intention or meaning behind their goal. In my experience, autistic/neurodivergent individuals appreciate clear, specific use of language, which supports them to see and reflect on what is in the spotlight. Additionally, many autistic/neurodivergent individuals notice, sometimes for the first time, their own proclivity for positive or negative self-expression, while collaboratively generating therapeutic goals.

Common goals for autistic/neurodivergent clients

As noted previously, there is no limit to the concerns that autistic/neurodivergent individuals may wish to pursue in therapy. As a point of interest only, the following is a short list of issues that multiple autistic/neurodivergent adults have cited in my practice as their motivation to seek therapy. Each of these would subsequently be collaboratively formed into a SMART goal, and an agreed-upon set of tasks established as a roadmap for therapy. Therapeutic tasks can become benchmarks for autistic/neurodivergent clients who are particularly drawn to monitoring their own progress in therapy. Individuals who avidly enjoy or rely upon categorization to support themselves in other areas of their lives, often find a similar process engaging and motivating, in therapy.

This list is provided with the intention of allowing neurotypical therapists to situate the concerns of their own neurodivergent clients within the context of the common concerns of the broader neurodivergent community. It is shared with gratitude to the autistic/neurodivergent individuals who have explored these, and many other concerns, in NAP with me:

1. Communication in important relationships
2. Unmasking or partially unmasking, in various contexts
3. Adult assessment and/or diagnosis of autism
4. Structure and routine in personal habits
5. Self-understanding/self-acceptance
6. Self-advocacy with intimate partners or friends
7. Self-advocacy in educational settings, with teachers/professors
8. Self-advocacy at work, with employers/clients/colleagues/HR departments
9. Neurodiversity-affirming parenting
10. Development of practical compensations for executive functioning issues
11. Understanding sensory processing and selfcare
12. Improved or structured conflict resolution techniques
13. Balancing selfcare with educational or career opportunities

While Ackerman and Hilsenroth (2001) proposed that a therapist's tendency to "over structure" therapy may negatively impact the therapeutic alliance, autistic/neurodivergent individuals often benefit from more structure and predictability in life in general. Many autistic individuals report a kind of cognitive freedom, arising from a clear understanding of how things work, or what is expected (by neurotypical individuals or systems), especially in new or unfamiliar settings. In the process of collaborative goal setting, the neurotypical therapist has the privilege of seeking an effective balance between providing enough structure and predictability that the autistic client feels safe and engaged with the process, but not so much as to preclude their opportunity to identify meaningful, personal therapeutic goals, while navigating the uncertainty the collaborative process itself may elicit. Here again, sufficient time needs to be spent establishing co-regulation between client and therapist before attempting collaboration to buffer against errors of judgement or pacing that may occur. If in doubt about the degree of structure needed, err on the side of suggesting too much, ask the client for input/feedback, and adjust accordingly.

Neuronormativity is pervasive in our culture, and messages of inferiority are equally damaging when they are subtle, embedded in systems, or quietly per-petuated in literature, as when they are verbally expressed. Change is inevitable, however, and therapists have daily opportunities to enact their social justice role within the therapy room. These opportunities arise naturally when collaborating on goal setting with autistic/neurodivergent clients. Careful attention is required to ensure that the goals we set together do not inadvertently perpetuate the idea that neurodivergence is the problem – this is our ethical responsibility, when supporting autistic/neurodivergent clients in psychotherapy.

Monitoring goals in NAP

Many clients gain encouragement and support from monitoring and discuss-ing their progress towards their therapeutic goals, once the goals and tasks are agreed on, and the journey begins. Similar to the heightened self-awareness that may emerge from the goal setting process, autistic/neurodivergent individuals often notice their own affinity for patterns and categorizing and identify them as strengths, while monitoring their progress toward goals. Autistic/neurodivergent individuals may benefit from a written set of their goals, to review and refer to as needed, or from a therapy notebook in which to record important moments or things they wish to discuss. Additionally, many autistic/neurodivergent clients appreciate a brief, ritualised "check-in" to create more predictability and struc-ture in their therapeutic experience, and monitoring goals provides a natural and positive opportunity for this.

Therapist growth and development

Clearly, the neurotypical therapist is holding a lot, in cross-neurotype psy-chotherapy – a lighter load than the new client is carrying, but a significant load nonetheless! This is an unfamiliar relational experience for many thera-pists and is not well-recognized nor supported yet by mainstream therapeutic approaches. Psychotherapy can be isolating work, even when client and ther-apist are neurologically aligned, or feel as if they are. In my experience, neu-rotypical therapists who are drawn to working in cross-neurotype alliances are special ones: compassionate, curious, inclusive, and deeply committed to mental health, writ large. They have hearts that deeply value relationship and connection between humans, and shoulders upon which they balance awareness of challenges such as distractibility or rapid overwhelm in the client, together with awareness of their own challenges with cross-neurotype communication, or limits placed upon their work by factors beyond their influence.

However, the cross-neurotype alliance is highly generative. Certainly, it emerges from the bond, the goals, and the tasks of psychotherapy, but it is not business as usual. It has a unique life force that attracts psychotherapists who are profoundly committed to client wellbeing, concerned with matters of social justice, and dedicated to their own personal and professional growth. And it attracts psychotherapists who are resilient, unwavering in their belief in healing through relationship, and dedicated to experiencing the journey, moment by moment. There is an authentic vibrancy and unique connectivity within the cross-neurotype therapeutic alliance, where great things can and do happen, for clients and therapists alike.

References

Ackerman, S. J., & Hilsenroth, M. J. (2001). A review of therapist characteristics and techniques negatively impacting the therapeutic alliance. *Psychotherapy: Theory, Research, Practice, Training, 38*(2), 171.

Bordin, E. S. (1979). The generalizability of the psychoanalytic concept of the working alliance. *Psychotherapy: Theory, Research & Practice, 16*(3), 252.

Bovend'Eerdt, T. J., Botell, R. E., & Wade, D. T. (2009). Writing SMART rehabilitation goals and achieving goal attainment scaling: A practical guide. *Clinical Rehabilitation, 23*(4), 352–361.

Camilleri, L. J., Maras, K., & Brosnan, M. (2024). Self-set goals: Autistic adults facilitating their self-determination through digitally mediated social stories. *Autism in Adulthood.* https://doi.org/10.1089/aut.2023.0063

Conoley, C. W., & Scheel, M. J. (2017). *Goal focused positive psychotherapy: A strengths-based approach.* Oxford University Press.

Cooper, M., & Dryden, W. (Eds.). (2015). *The handbook of pluralistic counselling and psychotherapy.* Sage.

De Shazer, S., Dolan, Y., Korman, H., Trepper, T., McCollum, E., & Berg, I. K. (2021). *More than miracles: The state of the art of solution-focused brief therapy.* Routledge.

Gable, S. (2006). Approach and avoidance social motives and goals. *Journal of Personality, 74*(1), 175–222.

Grandin, T., & Scariano, M. M. (1986). *Emergence: Labeled autistic.* Arena Press.

Grosse, M., & Grawe, K. (2002). Bern Inventory of treatment goals: Part 1. Development and first application of a taxonomy of treatment goal themes. *Psychotherapy Research, 12*(1), 79–99.

Hodgetts, S., Richards, K., & Park, E. (2018). Preparing for the future: Multi-stakeholder perspectives on autonomous goal setting for adolescents with autism spectrum disorders. *Disability and Rehabilitation, 40*(20), 2372–2379.

Holliday-Willey, L. (1999). *Pretending to be normal: Living with Asperger's syndrome.* Jessica Kingsley.

Kayrouz, R., & Hansen, S. (2020). I don't believe in miracles: Using the ecological validity model to adapt the miracle question to match the client's cultural preferences and characteristics. *Professional Psychology: Research and Practice, 51*(3), 223.

Chapter 10

Autism, attachment, and accessibility in Neurodiversity-Affirming Psychotherapy (NAP)

Autistic/neurodivergent individuals who seek mental health care frequently encounter a panoply of aversive environmental and social barriers limiting their access to accessible counselling and psychotherapy. The unacceptable consequences of this unequal access to appropriate care include significantly worse mental health among the autistic/neurodivergent population than the neurotypical, including documented higher incidence of self-harm and suicidality. Psychotherapists can take steps to address discriminatory healthcare practices, through their clinical work and in the wider health system. In the following pages, multiple pathways to accessible mental health care for autistic/neurodivergent individuals through NAP are proposed.

This chapter provides responses to the following clinical questions:

1. What does the research on *accessibility* in healthcare demonstrate about the experience of autistic/neurodivergent clients/patients in clinical settings?
2. How can clinicians *proactively* improve access to mental healthcare for neurodivergent individuals?
3. Discuss the evidence supporting the need for an *alternative framework* to assess security or insecurity in cross-neurotype attachment relationships?

Accessibility to healthcare

Neurodivergent individuals are more susceptible to both physical and mental health problems than neurotypicals, for known and unknown reasons. What is known, is that autistic people experience multiple, systemic barriers to accessing healthcare (Shaw et al., 2023). In NAP, it is recognized that many such barriers are attributable to the lack of recognition or accommodation of the communication, sensory, and executive functioning aspects of neurodivergence in clinical settings.

There is clear statistical evidence that healthcare in general is significantly less accessible to autistic individuals than to the allistic population (Adams et al., 2024; Hall et al., 2020; Mazurek et al., 2023). At the most obvious level,

DOI: 10.4324/9781003430476-10

there is a glaring disparity in life expectancy between autistic and allistic populations. Hirvikoski et al., 2016 demonstrated that autistic people without co-occurring cognitive disabilities have a life expectancy of 54 years (and 37 years, among those with co-occurring cognitive disabilities), compared to 74 years in the non-autistic population. Additional and compelling evidence of the disparity of access to mental healthcare was highlighted by Doherty et al. (2022), who identified suicide as the leading cause of death in the autistic population, with completed suicide nine times more likely among autistic males and 13 times more likely among autistic females, than among their neurotypical counterparts.

Three specific features of neurodivergence highlighted in this book have significant impacts on accessibility to physical and mental healthcare for autistic/neurodivergent individuals. Related to sensory processing, reduced interoception results in many autistic individuals having significantly increased pain tolerance, resulting in reduced ability to notice (along with a disinclination to report) pain, until it is debilitating or even life-threatening. Along with reduced interoception, aversive sensory environments in healthcare settings increase the barriers that neurodivergent individuals must navigate to access care; neurodivergent sensory processing makes the sounds, sights, and smells of healthcare settings intolerable for many autistic/neurodivergent individuals. The communication features of neurodivergence can make it difficult for autistic individuals to verbally report pain or other symptoms in ways that neurotypical clinicians understand, highlighting the double empathy problem (DEP) explained below (Milton, 2012). Executive functioning difficulties reduce the neurodivergent individual's capacity to navigate healthcare systems, from booking appointments, to managing competing demands on one's time and energy, to arranging coverage for work, kids, or pets to navigating transit or parking, to finding the location of a clinic within a large, unfamiliar setting, and so forth. Additionally, for systemic and personal reasons, the pace at which many neurotypical clinicians conduct appointments is often inaccessible to autistic/neurodivergent individuals, providing inadequate time or supports to process what has been said, to ask questions, and to process the experience meaningfully.

A tragic outcome of aversive healthcare environments and inaccessible interactions with clinicians and healthcare administrators is that autistic/neurodivergent individuals often avoid seeking healthcare until their illness or suffering becomes untenable, or even life threatening. As captured by Doherty et al., "Reduction of healthcare inequalities for autistic people requires that healthcare providers understand autistic perspectives, communication needs and sensory sensitivities. Adjustments for autism-specific [healthcare] needs are as necessary as ramps for wheelchair users" (2022, p. 1). In psychotherapy, with increased awareness, goodwill, and a degree of intentionality and creativity in clinicians and the settings in which they see clients, such alternatives can easily include provision of NAP, availability of AAC (Alternative and Augmentative Communication), and provision of viable alternatives to clinic-based care including such evidence-based modalities as virtual therapy, nature-based therapy, and animal-assisted therapy.

The Double (and Triple) Empathy Problem (DEP)

An important contribution to the literature highlights the communication breakdowns that often occur in cross-neurotype interactions. Given the high stakes, these are obviously pertinent in healthcare, but particularly in psychotherapy, where interpersonal communication is the main vehicle for treatment. Challenging the traditional medical model of autism as a problem within the individual, Milton (2012) widens the lens to appropriately place the issue of communication breakdown where it belongs: in the space between two individuals engaged (or trying to engage) in an interaction. Milton (2012) highlighted that individuals who have different experiences of the world are very likely to encounter difficulty in empathizing with one another, and that this may be further complicated by different language usage and comprehension, in both directions. Applied to clinical interactions, Milton's depiction of DEP illuminates the "disjuncture in reciprocity between two differently disposed social actors who hold different norms and expectations of each other, such as is common in autistic to non-autistic social interactions" (Milton, 2012, p. 884).

The DEP as it pertains to cross-neurotype interactions was investigated by Sheppard et al. (2023), exploring the nature of nominal "mindreading abilities" between neurodivergent and neurotypical individuals. Importantly, they demonstrated that interactions between two autistic individuals, or two non-autistic individuals, feature *similar degrees of interactional breakdown*; the DEP was observed only in interactions between individuals with different neurotypes, demonstrating a difference of empathy between two people rather than a deficiency (of empathy) in one of them. Furthering the discussion of the DEP into the realm of accessibility to healthcare for neurodivergent individuals, Shaw et al. (2023) examined how medical culture and language intensify the communication breakdowns that are common between autistic/neurodivergent individuals and healthcare practitioners. Their recognition of this additional layer of complexity highlights the triple empathy problem, calling attention to the systemic challenges faced by neurodivergent individuals in healthcare settings which place additional distance between autistic/neurodivergent individuals and the mental and physical healthcare they need.

Attachment theory

Secure attachment relationships emerge from regular, co-regulated interactions between parents and their babies. Fogel (1993, p. 28) describes co-regulation as a "continuous, mutual adaptation process", where parent and infant reach and sustain a state of "mutual social co-ordination" through responding to one another's actions, within a continuous feedback loop. There is a presupposition, however, that parents and babies attune to and adapt their shared rhythms and patterns with relative ease, perhaps reflecting an assumption that they have the same neurotype. In my experience, establishing co-regulation between a baby and parent that have different neurotypes differs slightly, requiring a higher degree of awareness and adaptation on the parent's part, to attune to the baby's internal rhythms and to learn to "dance" with them (Hughes, 2006, p. 3). Fortunately, most new parents are both endlessly creative and (almost!) tireless in their efforts to understand and respond to their baby's needs and messages. Certainly, co-regulation happens across neurotypes; it generally takes a little longer, and requires a touch more creativity, than neurotypical parents usually anticipate!

The concept of co-regulation matters greatly to our understanding of secure attachment patterns and behaviours within relationships, and it matters just as much to our conceptualization of NAP as attachment-based, cross-neurotype psychotherapy. Co-regulation underlies the formation of a secure attachment relationship between parent and infant, which becomes a template for the baby's future relational experiences. In contrast, individuals whose earliest relationships were not co-regulated, and did not result in secure attachment, often experience a repeating pattern of relational difficulties, accompanied by associated mental health impacts: loneliness, anxiety, depression and so forth. In the context of early life relational trauma, Hughes et al. referred to the critical developmental role of co-regulation, emphasizing that "young children need these synchronized nonverbal – and gradually verbal – interactions that are part of healthy caregiving in order to develop neurologically, emotionally, socially and cognitively" (2019, p. 4).

Baumeister and Leary (1995) proposed that attachment theory is rooted in the fact that humans need to connect with one another, and that interpersonal relationships are the basis for security, acceptance, and a sense of belonging. And, unless they intentionally decide to do otherwise parents generally interact with their infants (and young children) in ways that reflect how they were parented; on a basic level, those who experienced co-regulation as infants, are usually well-positioned to establish it with their own baby, many years later.

Attachment and autism

In early life relationships between neurotypical babies and neurotypical parents, safety and reciprocity in infant-parent interactions are the relational experiences from which secure attachment relationships develop. Both safety and reciprocity are expressed and experienced through frequent, mutually enjoyable, co-regulated interactions. And in the absence of extenuating circumstances, parents and babies who are attuned to one another engage in such interactions with relative ease.

Cross-neurotype co-regulation may not be quite so straightforward. A neurodivergent parent may have difficulty interpreting and attuning to their neurotypical infant's need for reciprocity, for example, and it is equally plausible that a neurotypical parent may have similar difficulties attuning to their neurodivergent baby's needs. In the neuronormative parenting culture, it is not difficult to imagine which of these parents would be likely to receive extensive support within and beyond the healthcare system, and which is likely to be questioned, criticized, or judged for their parenting style, predisposing them to anxiety and other mental health difficulties, and even to relational strain between themselves and their infant.

I am not suggesting that secure attachment does not develop in cross-neurotype relationships; it clearly does! What I am suggesting is that it would be helpful and indeed timely, to explore whether our current understanding of secure attachment, as articulated by (Ainsworth et al., 1978; Bowlby, 1969, 1979; Main, 1996) is spacious enough to identify and include cross-neurotype secure attachment. Perhaps it is, but if it is not (and our currently available assessment tools don't accurately assess cross-neurotype attachment relationships) we are at risk of continuing to pathologize autistic ways of being in relationship. It would be ironic indeed if attachment theory and attachment-based clinical practices were found to inadvertently promote neuronormativity. Clinically, it seems reasonable to propose that there is space to assess cross-neurotype attachment styles, and to do so differently from how we assess attachment relationships between parents and babies whose neurotypes align. Clearly, research is indicated, and neurodiversity-affirming assessment tools are needed, in this area of developmental psychology and infant mental health.

Secure attachment in autism

Teague et al. (2017, p. 35) found ample evidence in the literature supporting the development of secure attachment behaviour in autistic children, including the classic behaviours of seeking safety with parents when distressed and using parents as a secure base when exploring. They also highlighted the caregivers' way of being, and their own internal working model of caregiving, as impactful on the quality of the attachment. As previously mentioned, the DEP (Milton, 2012) is consistently noted only in interactions between individuals with different neurotypes, and interactions between two autistic individuals (or two non-autistic individuals) feature comparable degrees of interactional breakdown. From an attachment perspective, this illuminates the possibility that an autistic/neurodivergent parent may co-regulate more easily with an autistic/neurodivergent baby, setting the groundwork for a classically defined, secure attachment rela-tionship. This idea was anecdotally supported in a recent conversation with an autistic adult, who opined that masking is not specific to the autistic experience, noting correctly that that most humans adapt in certain ways to social situations. Significantly, this autistic/neurodivergent individual was raised by neurodi-vergent parents, within a neurodiversity-affirming family and home in which nobody masked. It seems reasonable therefore, to propose that neurodivergence in parents may facilitate a secure attachment relationship between them and their neurodivergent baby, at least more easily than for a cross-neurotype parent-baby team!

The obvious, practical question is whether it is possible, or even desirable, for new parents to muse about whether they and their infant have the same or differ-ent neurotypes. In my experience, most new parents are too busy rocking, sing-ing, nursing, or gazing in wonderment while questioning if they will ever get to shower again … to be concerned with such matters. However, psychotherapists do have the option of observing and exploring whether they and their clients have the same or different neurotypes, and reflecting on how they will provide an accessible, co-regulated therapeutic experience, considering whatever they recognize. In doing so, they significantly increase the likelihood of successfully working with a client whose neurotype differs from their own, establishing trust and moving towards a stronger therapeutic alliance and positive therapeutic out-comes, in the process.

Cross-neurotype, attachment-based therapy

Trust between parent and child is foundational for the formation of secure attachment (Bowlby, 1969). Attachment-based therapies are therefore aligned with the position that trust is integral to healthy relationships (Crits-Christoph et al., 2019), including the relationship between client and therapist. The work-ing alliance must be based upon mutual trust for therapy to have positive out-comes. However, trust is a complex issue in therapy, encompassing more than the familiar questions of client confidentiality, public safety, and systemic accountability – and additionally so in cross-neurotype therapeutic alliances.

Consideration of trust within the therapeutic alliance requires acknowledg-ment and careful handling of the balance of power in the relationship. Traditional models of therapy, psychoanalytic and behavioural alike, placed most of the power in the therapist's hands, positioning them as the authority on what is healthy, advisable, or otherwise. When things went well, this power imbalance allowed therapists to exaggerate their contribution to the outcomes, diminishing the client's role accordingly. Conversely, when things went poorly, this unequal distribution of power enabled therapists to defer responsibility for therapeutic rupture onto the client, often perpetuating the individual's negative perception of themselves and their role in relational breakdown outside of therapy. Post-modern therapeutic frameworks appropriately challenge this dynamic; feminist, narrative, and social justice therapeutic models among others, have redistributed power in the therapeutic alliance, such that both client and therapist are co-creating the process, constructing the framework for desired change, and sharing the responsibility for (or celebration of) the outcomes.

McNamee (2009, p. 57) articulated that a post-modern therapeutic framework shifts the focus "away from centering individuals and their actions" towards "centering processes of relating." While this is the desired direction for NAP, many autistic/neurodivergent adults have had minimal or tokenistic experience with self-determination from childhood onward. These individuals may initially have legitimate difficulty enacting their role as a co-creator of the process, requiring additional time and regular experiences of co-regulated interactions within the therapeutic alliance, to risk doing so. This points to the therapist's responsibility to regularly assess and reflect on the power dynamic in the alliance; to solicit and integrate client feedback throughout the process; to seek clinical and peer supervision on areas of concern or growth; and to pause and address any imbalance of power that arises. And in the therapeutic alliance between a neurodivergent client and a neurotypical therapist, this responsibility is magnified by the impacts of neuronormativity upon both individuals, upon the therapeutic setting, upon the culture of mental healthcare, and upon the wider culture within which this therapeutic alliance is situated.

One of the most damaging neuronormative misconceptions of autism/neurodivergence is that autistic individuals do not need nor even want, friends and relationships. This ridiculous notion has been repeatedly refuted by autistic/neurodivergent clients in my practice and is echoed in every corner of the neurodivergent community online. Crompton et al. (2020) demonstrated that autistic individuals regularly describe feelings of ease and comfort when socializing with other autistic individuals, further supporting the position that co-regulation between individuals with the same neurotype is easier to establish than cross-neurotype co-regulation. This highlights two important points: one is that autistic people are often lonely in the dominant culture and may benefit in therapy from support and encouragement to connect with others in the autistic/neurodivergent community. The other is that there is a significant need for autistic/neurodivergent therapists in the profession, who are uniquely qualified and naturally inclined to provide NAP to autistic/neurodivergent clients.

Holding jello and other concerns

Chapman (2020, p. 220) drew attention to neurodiversity as "a call to alter how we have so far failed to empathize with neurological others, as well as how to design public spaces and scientific experiments". NAP proposes pathways by which neurotypical psychotherapists may respond to this call. These responses include self-awareness, self-care, and reflective practice; competency in providing autistic/neurodivergent clients with accessible, attachment-based psychotherapy; willingness to support clients to self-advocate when needed; and courage to advocate within the therapist's own clinical setting and beyond, for increased access to neurodiversity-affirming healthcare services.

A wonderfully articulate autistic client in my practice uses the analogy of "holding jello" to describe moments of great uncertainty; those moments when one is aware that something important is happening, but it is not clear which pieces of the experience should be held onto, and which may be released without significant consequences. Incidentally, this individual really enjoys jello, and their deeper conviction is that no part of such a delicious and slippery handful can be easily released! Writing this book has been remarkably like holding jello; it has been bigger (and a bit messier) than I anticipated, and as it concludes, knowing what to do with, or about, the pieces I have had to release, is more challenging than anticipated. There are many important topics that regularly arise in therapy with neurodivergent individuals, that have not been addressed in this book, regrettably. However, excellent frameworks for NAP are emerging in many settings, and all kinds of minds are needed to explore and develop it, to bolster the evidence base, and to carry neurodiversity-affirming clinical strategies forward.

For the particular attention of psychotherapists providing NAP, some of those "released" topics include gender dysphoria, gender fluidity, body dysmorphia, and disordered eating (especially avoidant/restrictive food intake disorder [ARFID]). Currently, neurodiversity-affirming professional learning opportunities are inadequate, and the need is great.

Among researchers, significant work is needed around cross-neurotype attachment relationships across the lifespan. The incidence of relationship breakdown where one partner is neurodivergent and the other neurotypical is highly distressing, and factors that support and sustain cross-neurotype relationships have yet to be clearly identified. Developing informed frameworks for supporting secure attachment in neurodivergent families, and for working with cross-neurotype couples, are pressing concerns. Additionally, as proposed earlier, development of measurement tools to accurately assess cross-neurotype attachment styles are needed, for both adult and parent-child relationships, from which evidence-based neurodiversity-affirming parenting and relationship supports and interventions may be developed.

Shaw et al. (2023) highlighted the need for autism training in medical curricula, providing solid recommendations for best practices in providing healthcare services for autistic individuals. A cultural shift is required to continue to support and encourage interdisciplinary collaboration, and to do so in ways that are truly accessible to neurodivergent clients/patients, clinicians, and researchers. Shaw et al. (2023) also spotlight the need for more autistic doctors in the medical workforce; the identical need is a pressing concern in psychotherapy. Neurodivergent psychotherapists, proportionate to the prevalence of neurodivergent individuals in the population, are urgently needed, and effective ways of supporting these individuals to enter the counselling/psychotherapy profession and to safely navigate the demands of study/training, require identification and provision.

Addressing clinical gaps requires clinical training programs to self-examine regarding accessibility to neurodivergent learners; currently, the pacing and communication-related expectations of training in psychotherapy (and in medicine) discriminates against individuals who take in and process information in neurodivergent ways. Similarly, the communication, sensory processing, and executive functioning aspects of neurodivergence regularly cause untenable additional stress for neurodivergent learners striving to succeed within neuronormative academic practices, such as group-based or collaborative projects, peer assessment, standards-based grading, and timed examinations.

Neurodivergent clinicians bring unique sensitivities and capacity for caring to their work with clients and patients. Autistic/neurodivergent high school students who are inclined to enter the helping professions therefore need informed support to do so; currently, the pervasive automatic response of the educational system is to direct (or redirect) autistic/neurodivergent students into science, technology, engineering, and mathematics (STEM) fields, because of their diagnosis and often regardless of their stated personal goals and interests. There is clearly an urgent need for informed advocacy and awareness of neurodivergence, and around neurodiversity in general, throughout the educational and healthcare systems, and beyond.

Where do we go from here? Who should we ask for directions?

A map is a very good way to get to a destination, or at least to be assured we are headed in the right direction. Many autistic/neurodivergent individuals, from early childhood and throughout their lives, are intrepid explorers and those who have a particular interest in cartography are usually a step (or several) ahead of neurotypicals, when it comes to creating, reading, or following a map. Therefore, when we come to a juncture in work or life, and we are wondering which direction to turn, it is often wise to pause and ask an autistic/neurodivergent individual for directions. In neurodiversity-affirming clinical work, my experience is that many autistic/neurodivergent individuals already know where we need to go next, and how we might get there. Cross-neurotype, consultation and collaboration in mental healthcare will enable us to move forward with clarity, and insight, on the journey to providing neurodiversity-affirming psychotherapy, and far beyond. And if you sometimes feel lost, pause, and ask your autistic client which way to go. You will find the path, if you are brave enough to look for it together.

Clinicians, instructors, and clinical supervisors are welcome to use or adapt the following questions as springboards for learning in clinical supervision, professional teaching and development, or reflective practice:

1. What do I know/believe about the function and distribution of power within the therapeutic alliance?
2. How do I hold my share of the power in cross-neurotype psychotherapy? How do I actively ensure that autistic/neurodivergent clients can safely take up theirs?
3. What does a neurodiversity-affirming therapeutic space look and feel like?
4. Who can I invite into the therapeutic space to provide feedback on accessibility for NAP?
5. What assumptions need to be made explicit in the therapeutic space, to ensure an appropriate balance of power between autistic/neurodivergent clients and me?
6. What is the evidence that supports the demand for neurodiversity-affirming clinical practice, and equitable access to mental healthcare?

References

Adams, N., Jacobsen, K., Li, L., Francino, M., Rutherford, L., Tei, C., Scheim, A., & Bauer, G. (2024). Health and health care access of autistic transgender and nonbinary people in Canada: A cross-sectional study. *Autism in Adulthood.* https://doi.org/10.1089/aut.2023.0024

Ainsworth, M. D. S., Blehar, M. C., Waters, E., & Wall, S. (1978). *Patterns of attachment: A psychological study of the strange situation.* Lawrence Erlbaum.

Baumeister, R., & Leary, M. (1995). The need to belong: Desire for interpersonal attachments as a fundamental human motivation. *Psychological Bulletin, 117,* 497–529.

Bowlby, J. (1969). *Attachment and loss: Vol. 1 Attachment.* Basic Books.

Bowlby, J. (1979). The Bowlby-Ainsworth attachment theory. *Behavioral and Brain Sciences, 2*(4), 637–638.

Chapman, R. (2020). Defining neurodiversity for research and practice. In H. Rosqvist, N. Chown & A. Stenning (Eds.), *Neurodiversity studies* (pp. 218–220). Routledge.

Crits-Christoph, P., Rieger, A., Gaines, A., & Gibbons, M. B. C. (2019). Trust and respect in the patient-clinician relationship: Preliminary development of a new scale. *BMC Psychology, 7,* 1–8.

Crompton, C. J., Hallett, S., Ropar, D., Flynn, E., & Fletcher-Watson, S. (2020). 'I never realised everybody felt as happy as I do when I am around autistic people': A thematic analysis of autistic adults' relationships with autistic and neurotypical friends and family. *Autism, 24*(6), 1438–1448.

Doherty, M., Neilson, S., O'Sullivan, J., Carravallah, L., Johnson, M., Cullen, W., & Shaw, S. C. (2022). Barriers to healthcare and self-reported adverse outcomes for autistic adults: A cross-sectional study. *BMJ Open, 12*(2), e056904.

Fogel, A. (1993). *Developing through relationships*. University of Chicago Press.

Hall, J. P., Batza, K., Streed, C. G., Boyd, B. A., & Kurth, N. K. (2020). Health disparities among sexual and gender minorities with autism spectrum disorder. *Journal of Autism and Developmental DisordersDisorders, 50*(8), 3071–3077.

Hirvikoski, T., Mittendorfer-Rutz, E., Boman, M., Larsson, H., Lichtenstein, P., & Bölte, S. (2016). Premature mortality in autism spectrum disorder. *The British Journal of Psychiatry, 208*(3), 232–238.

Hughes, D. A. (2006). *Building the bonds of attachment: Awakening love in deeply troubled children*. Jason Aronson.

Hughes, D. A., Golding, K. S., & Hudson, J. (2019). *Healing relational trauma with attachment-focused interventions: Dyadic developmental psychotherapy with children and families*. WW Norton & Company.

Main, M. (1996). Introduction to the special section on attachment and psychopathology: 2. Overview of the field of attachment. *Journal of Consulting and Clinical Psychology, 64*(2), 237–243. https://doi.org/10.1037/0022-006X.64.2.237

Mazurek, M. O., Sadikova, E., Cheak-Zamora, N., Hardin, A., Sohl, K., & Malow, B. A. (2023). Health care needs, experiences, and perspectives of autistic adults. *Autism in Adulthood, 5*(1), 51–62.

McNamee, S. (2009). Postmodern psychotherapeutic ethics: Relational responsibility in practice. *Human Systems: The Journal of Therapy, Consultation & Training, 20*(1), 57–71.

Milton, D. E. (2012). On the ontological status of autism: The 'double empathy problem'. *Disability & Society, 27*(6), 883–887.

Shaw, S. C., Carravallah, L., Johnson, M., O'Sullivan, J., Chown, N., Neilson, S., & Doherty, M. (2023). Barriers to healthcare and a 'triple empathy problem' may lead to adverse outcomes for autistic adults: A qualitative study. *Autism: the international journal of research and practice, 13623613231205629. Advance online publication.* https://doi.org/10.1177/13623613231205629

Sheppard, E., Webb, S., & Wilkinson, H. (2023). Mindreading beliefs in same-and cross-neurotype interactions. *Autism, 18,,* 13623613231211456.

Teague, S. J., Gray, K. M., Tonge, B. J., & Newman, L. K. (2017). Attachment in children with autism spectrum disorder: A systematic review. *Research in Autism Spectrum Disorders, 35*, 35–50.

Bibliography

Ackerman, S. J., & Hilsenroth, M. J. (2001). A review of therapist characteristics and techniques negatively impacting the therapeutic alliance. *Psychotherapy: Theory, Research, Practice, Training, 38*(2), 171.

Adams, D., & Young, K. (2021). A systematic review of the perceived barriers and facilitators to accessing psychological treatment for mental health problems in individuals on the autism spectrum. *Review Journal of Autism and Developmental Disorders, 8*(4), 436–453.

Adams, N., Jacobsen, K., Li, L., Francino, M., Rutherford, L., Tei, C., Scheim, A., & Bauer, G. (2024). Health and health care access of autistic transgender and nonbinary people in Canada: A cross-sectional study. *Autism in Adulthood.* https://doi.org/10.1089/aut.2023.0024

Adler, A. (1928). *Die Technik der individual-Psychologie.* Bergmann.

Ainsworth, M. D. S., Blehar, M. C., Waters, E., & Wall, S. (1978). *Patterns of attachment: A psychological study of the strange situation.* Lawrence Erlbaum.

Amaral, D., Geschwind, D., & Dawson, G. (Eds.). (2011). *Autism spectrum disorders.* Oxford University Press.

American Psychiatric Association. (2022). *Diagnostic and statistical manual of mental disorders.* American Psychiatric Association. https://doi.org/10.1176/APPI.BOOKS.9780890425596

Anagnostou, E., Zwaigenbaum, L., Szatmari, P., Fombonne, E., Fernandez, B. A., Woodbury-Smith, M., Brian, J., Bryson, S., Smith, I. M., Drmic, I., Buchanan, J. A., Roberts, W., & Scherer, S. W. (2014). Autism spectrum disorder: Advances in evidence-based practice. *Canadian Medical Association Journal, 186*(7), 509–519.

Anda, R. F., Brown, D. W., Dube, S. R., Bremner, J. D., Felitti, V. J., & Giles, W. H. (2008). Adverse childhood experiences and chronic obstructive pulmonary disease in adults. *American Journal of Preventive Medicine, 34*(5), 396–403. https://doi.org/10.1016/J.AMEPRE.2008.02.002

Andresen, R., Oades, L., & Caputi, P. (2003). The experience of recovery from schizophrenia: Towards an empirically-validated stage model. *Australian and New Zealand Journal of Psychiatry, 37*, 586–594.

Arnold, S. R., Higgins, J. M., Weise, J., Desai, A., Pellicano, E., & Trollor, J. N. (2023). Confirming the nature of autistic burnout. *Autism, 20*(7), 1906–1918.

Aron, E. N. (2013). *The highly sensitive person: How to thrive when the world over-whelms you*. Kensington Publishing.

Attwood, T. (1998). *Asperger's syndrome: A guide for parents and professionals*. Jessica Kingsley Publications.

Attwood, T. (2003). Understanding and managing circumscribed interests. In M. Prior (Ed.), *Learning and behavior problems in Asperger syndrome* (pp. 126–147). The Guilford Press.

Audet, C., & Paré, D. (2017). Social justice and counseling: Discourse in practice. *Social Justice and Counseling: Discourse in Practice*, 1–262. https://doi.org/10.4324/978131 5753751

Au-Yeung, S. K., Bradley, L., Robertson, A. E., Shaw, R., Baron-Cohen, S., & Cassidy, S. (2019). Experience of mental health diagnosis and perceived misdiagnosis in autistic, possibly autistic and non-autistic adults. *Autism*, *23*(6), 1508–1518.

Ayres, A. J. (1972). Improving academic scores through sensory integration. *Journal of Learning Disabilities*, *5*(6), 338–343.

Ayers, A. J. (2005). *Sensory integration and the child*. Western Psychological Services.

Baldwin, M. (2013). *The use of self in therapy*. Routledge. www.routledge.com/The-Use-of-Self-in-Therapy/Baldwin/p/book/9780415896030

Ball, B., Sevillano, L., Faulkner, M., & Belseth, T. (2021). Agency, genuine support, and emotional connection: Experiences that promote relational permanency in foster care. *Children and Youth Services Review*, *121*, 105852.

Baron-Cohen, S. (2008). *Autism and Asperger syndrome*. OUP Oxford.

Barrett, A. C. (2020). *Symptom presentation of children with autism spectrum disorder after adverse childhood experiences*. University of California.

Baudino, L. M. (2010). Autism spectrum disorder: A case of misdiagnosis. *American Journal of Dance Therapy*, *32*(2), 113–129.

Baumeister, R., & Leary, M. (1995). The need to belong: Desire for interpersonal attachments as a fundamental human motivation. *Psychological Bulletin*, *117*, 497–529.

Baumeister, R. F., & Leary, M. R. (2017). The need to belong: Desire for interpersonal attachments as a fundamental human motivation. *Interpersonal Development*, 57–89.

Bauminger, N., & Kasari, C. (2000). Loneliness and friendship in high-functioning children with autism. *Child Development*, *71*(2), 447–456. https://doi.org/10.1111/1467-8624.00156

Benamer, S., & White, K. (2018). *Trauma and attachment*. Routledge.

Benavides-Rawson, J., & Grinker, R. R. (2018). Reactive attachment disorder and autism spectrum disorder: Diagnosis and care in a cultural context. In *Trauma, Autism, and Neurodevelopmental Disorders: Integrating Research, Practice, and Policy* (pp. 149–160).

Benford, P., & Standen, P. J. (2009). The Internet: A comfortable communication medium for autistic people? *Journal of Assistive Technologies*, *3*(2), 44–53.

Bettelheim, B. (1967). *The empty fortress: Infantile autism and the birth of the self*. Free Press of Glencoe.

Billeiter, K. B., & Froiland, J. M. (2023). Diversity of intelligence is the norm within the autism spectrum: Full scale intelligence scores among children with ASD. *Child Psychiatry & Human Development, 54*, 1094–1101.

Bordin, E. S. (1979). The generalizability of the psychoanalytic concept of the working alliance. *Psychotherapy: Theory, Research & Practice, 16*(3), 252.

Botha, M., Dibb, B., & Frost, D. M. (2022). "Autism is me": An investigation of how autistic individuals make sense of autism and stigma. *Disability and Society, 37*(3), 427–453. https://doi.org/10.1080/09687599.2020.1822782

Bottema-Beutel, K., Kapp, S. K., Lester, J. N., Sasson, N. J., & Hand, B. N. (2021). Avoiding ableist language: Suggestions for autism researchers. *Autism in Adulthood, 3*(1).

Boullier, M., & Blair, M. (2018). Adverse childhood experiences. *Paediatrics and Child Health, 28*(3), 132–137. https://doi.org/10.1016/J.PAED.2017.12.008

Bovend'Eerdt, T. J., Botell, R. E., & Wade, D. T. (2009). Writing SMART rehabilitation goals and achieving goal attainment scaling: A practical guide. *Clinical Rehabilitation, 23*(4), 352–361.

Bowlby, J. (1969). *Attachment and loss: Vol. 1 attachment*. Basic Books.

Bowlby, J. (1979). The Bowlby-Ainsworth attachment theory. *Behavioral and Brain Sciences, 2*(4), 637–638.

Bowlby, J. (1988). *A secure base: Parent-child attachment and healthy human development*. Basic Books.

Brookman-Frazee, L., Drahota, A., Stadnick, N., & Palinkas, L. A. (2012). Therapist perspectives on community mental health services for children with autism spectrum disorders. *Administration and Policy in Mental Health, 39*(5), 365. https://doi.org/10.1007/S10488-011-0355-Y

Brown, C., & Dunn, W. (2002). *Adolescent/adult sensory profile*. Psychological Corporation.

Bryan, L. C., & Gast, D. L. (2000). Teaching on-task and on-schedule behaviors to high-functioning children with autism via picture activity schedules. *Journal of Autism and Developmental Disorders, 30*(6), 553–567. https://doi.org/10.1023/A:1005687310346

Bucci, S., Seymour-Hyde, A., Harris, A., & Berry, K. (2016). Client and therapist attachment styles and working alliance. *Clinical Psychology & Psychotherapy, 23*(2), 155–165.

Burke, E., Danquah, A., & Berry, K. (2016). A qualitative exploration of the use of attachment theory in adult psychological therapy. *Clinical Psychology and Psychotherapy, 23*(2), 142–154. https://doi.org/10.1002/CPP.1943

Butler, L. D., Critelli, F. M., & Rinfrette, E. S. (2011). Trauma-informed care and mental health. *Directions in Psychiatry, 31*(3), 197–212.

Cage, E., di Monaco, J., & Newell, V. (2018). Experiences of autism acceptance and mental health in autistic adults. *Journal of Autism and Developmental Disorders, 48*, 473–484.

Cain, S. (2013). *Quiet: The power of introverts in a world that can't stop talking*. Crown.

Camilleri, L. J., Maras, K., & Brosnan, M. (2024). *Self-set goals: Autistic adults facilitating their self-determination through digitally mediated social stories*. Autism in Adulthood.

Canadian Counselling and Psychotherapy Association. (2021). *Standards of practice* (6th ed.). CCPA.

Cappadocia, M. C., Weiss, J. A., & Pepler, D. (2012). Bullying experiences among children and youth with Autism Spectrum Disorders. *Journal of Autism and Developmental Disorders, 42*, 266–277.

Cassidy, S. A., Gould, K., Townsend, E., Pelton, M., Robertson, A. E., & Rodgers, J. (2020). Is camouflaging autistic traits associated with suicidal thoughts and behaviours? Expanding the interpersonal psychological theory of suicide in an undergraduate student sample. *Journal of Autism and Developmental Disorders, 50*, 3638–3648.

Cassidy, S., Bradley, L., Shaw, R., & Baron-Cohen, S. (2018). Risk markers for suicidality in autistic adults. *Molecular Autism, 9*, 1–14.

Cassidy, S., Bradley, P., Robinson, J., Allison, C., McHugh, M., & Baron-Cohen, S. (2014). Suicidal ideation and suicide plans or attempts in adults with Asperger's syndrome attending a specialist diagnostic clinic: A clinical cohort study. *The Lancet Psychiatry, 1*(2), 142–147.

Chapman, L., Rose, K., Hull, L., & Mandy, W. (2022). "I want to fit in… but I don't want to change myself fundamentally": A qualitative exploration of the relationship between masking and mental health for autistic teenagers. *Research in Autism Spectrum Disorders, 99*, 102069.

Chapman, R. (2020). Defining neurodiversity for research and practice. In H. Rosqvist, N. Chown, & A. Stenning (Eds.), *Neurodiversity studies* (pp. 218–220). Routledge.

Charman, T., Pickles, A., Simonoff, E., Chandler, S., Loucas, T., & Baird, G. (2011). IQ in children with autism spectrum disorders: Data from the Special Needs and Autism Project (SNAP). *Psychological Medicine, 41*(3), 619–627. https://doi.org/10.1017/S0033291710000991

Clark, C. J., Liu, B. S., Winegard, B. M., & Ditto, P. H. (2019). Tribalism is human nature. *Current Directions in Psychological Science, 28*(6), 587–592. https://doi.org/10.1177/0963721419862289

Classen, C. C., & Clark, C. S. (2017). Trauma-informed care. In S. N. Gold (Ed.), *APA handbook of trauma psychology: Trauma practice* (pp. 515–541). American Psychological Association.

Cohen, K. R., Lee, C. M., & McIlwraith, R. (2012). The psychology of advocacy and the advocacy of psychology. *Canadian Psychology/Psychologie Canadienne, 53*(3), 151.

Collins, S., & Arthur, N. (2017). Challenging conversations: Deepening personal and professional commitment to culture-infused and socially just counselling practices. In C. Audet & D. Paré (Eds.), *Social Justice and Counseling: Discourse in Practice* (1st ed.). Routledge.

Comber, C. (2023). *The intersection of loneliness and counselling from a pluralistic perspective, using a hermeneutic approach* [Doctoral Dissertation]. ResearchSpace@ Auckland.

Conine, D. E., Campau, S. C., & Petronelli, A. K. (2022). LGBTQ+ conversion therapy and applied behavior analysis: A call to action. *Journal of Applied Behavior Analysis, 55*(1), 6–18. https://doi.org/10.1002/JABA.876

Connell, J., Grant, S., & Mullin, T. (2006). Client initiated termination of therapy at NHS primary care counselling services. *Counselling and Psychotherapy Research, 6*(1), 60–67.

Conoley, C. W., & Scheel, M. J. (2017). *Goal focused positive psychotherapy: A strengths-based approach*. Oxford University Press.

Cook, J., Hull, L., Crane, L., & Mandy, W. (2021). Camouflaging in autism: A systematic review. *Clinical Psychology Review*, *89*, 102080.

Cooper, M., & Dryden, W. (Eds.). (2015). *The handbook of pluralistic counselling and psychotherapy*. Sage.

Copeland, W. E., Wolke, D., Angold, A., & Costello, E. J. (2013). Adult psychiatric outcomes of bullying and being bullied by peers in childhood and adolescence. *JAMA Psychiatry*, *70*(4), 419–426. https://doi.org/10.1001/JAMAPSYCHIATRY.2013.504

Corey, G. (2013). *Theory and practice of counseling and psychotherapy* (9th ed.). Cengage Learning/Brooks Cole.

Cozolino, L. J., & Santos, E. N. (2014). Why we need therapy-and why it works: A neuroscientific perspective. *Smith College Studies in Social Work*, *84*(2–3), 157–177. https://doi.org/10.1080/00377317.2014.923630

Cravener, P. (1992). Establishing therapeutic alliance across cultural barriers. *Journal of Psychosocial Nursing and Mental Health Services*, *30*(12), 10–14. https://doi.org/10.3928/0279-3695-19921201-05

Crenshaw, K. (2013). Demarginalizing the intersection of race and sex: A black feminist critique of antidiscrimination doctrine, feminist theory and antiracist politics. In K. Maschke (Ed.), *Feminist legal theories* (pp. 23–51). Routledge.

Crethar, H. C., & Ratts, M. J. (2008). Why social justice is a counseling concern. *Counseling Today*, *50*(12), 24–25.

Crits-Christoph, P., Rieger, A., Gaines, A., & Gibbons, M. B. C. (2019). Trust and respect in the patient-clinician relationship: Preliminary development of a new scale. *BMC Psychology*, *7*, 1–8.

Croen, L. A., Zerbo, O., Qian, Y., Massolo, M. L., Rich, S., Sidney, S., & Kripke, C. (2015). The health status of adults on the autism spectrum. *Autism*, *19*(7), 814–823.

Crompton, C. J., Hallett, S., Ropar, D., Flynn, E., & Fletcher-Watson, S. (2020). 'I never realised everybody felt as happy as I do when I am around autistic people': A thematic analysis of autistic adults' relationships with autistic and neurotypical friends and family. *Autism*, *24*(6), 1438–1448.

Crowell, J. A., & Waters, E. (1994). Bowlby's theory grown up: The role of attachment in adult love relationships. *Psychological Inquiry*, *5*(1), 31–34. https://doi.org/10.1207/S15327965PLI0501_4

Davidson, C., Moran, H., & Minnis, H. (2022). Autism and attachment disorders – How do we tell the difference? *BJPsych Advances*, *28*(6), 371–380. https://doi.org/10.1192/BJA.2022.2

Davidson, L., Sells, D., Songster, S., & O'Connell, M. (2005). Qualitative studies of recovery: What can we learn from the person? In R. O. Ralph & P. W. Corrigan (Eds.), *Recovery in Mental Illness: Broadening Our Understanding of Wellness*, (pp. 147–170). American Psychological Association. https://doi.org/10.1037/10848-007

Davies, J., Glinn, L., Osborne, L. A., & Reed, P. (2023). Exploratory study of parenting differences for autism spectrum disorder and attachment disorder. *Journal of Autism and Developmental Disorders*, *53*(5), 2143–2152. https://doi.org/10.1007/S10803-022-05531-0

de Clercq, H., Jordan, R., Hume, K., & Roberts, J. (2019). Analysis of what makes a successful professional in autism. In *The SAGE handbook of autism and education*. Sage.

de Shazer, S., Dolan, Y., Korman, H., Trepper, T., McCollum, E., & Berg, I. K. (2021). *More than miracles: The state of the art of solution-focused brief therapy*. Routledge.

Degnan, A., Seymour-Hyde, A., Harris, A., & Berry, K. (2016). The role of therapist attachment in alliance and outcome: A systematic literature review. *Clinical Psychology & Psychotherapy*, *23*(1), 47–65.

DeLeon, P. H., Loftis, C. W., Ball, V., & Sullivan, M. J. (2006). Navigating politics, policy, and procedure: A firsthand perspective of advocacy on behalf of the profession. *Professional Psychology: Research and Practice*, *37*(2), 146.

Demetriou, E. A., Lampit, A., Quintana, D. S., Naismith, S. L., Song, Y. J. C., Pye, J. E., Hickie, I., & Guastella, A. J. (2018). Autism spectrum disorders: A meta-analysis of executive function. *Molecular Psychiatry*, *23*(5), 1198–1204. https://doi.org/10.1038/mp.2017.75

Diamond, A. (2013). Executive functions. *Annual Review of Psychology*, *64*, 135–168. https://doi.org/10.1146/ANNUREV-PSYCH-113011-143750

Dietz, P. M., Rose, C. E., McArthur, D., & Maenner, M. (2020). National and state estimates of adults with autism spectrum disorder. *Journal of Autism and Developmental Disorders*, *50*, 4258–4266.

Dill, B. T., & Kohlman, M. H. (2012). Intersectionality: A transformative paradigm in feminist theory and social justice. *Handbook of Feminist Research: Theory and Praxis*, *2*, 154–174.

Dodds, R. L. (2021). An exploratory review of the associations between adverse experiences and autism. *Journal of Aggression, Maltreatment & Trauma*, *30*(8), 1093–1112. https://doi.org/10.1080/10926771.2020.1783736

Doherty, M., Neilson, S., O'Sullivan, J., Carravallah, L., Johnson, M., Cullen, W., & Shaw, S. C. (2022). Barriers to healthcare and self-reported adverse outcomes for autistic adults: A cross-sectional study. *BMJ Open*, *12*(2), e056904.

Doige, N. (2007). *The brain that changes itself: Stories of personal triumph from the frontiers of brain science*. Penguin.

Doove, B. M., Feron, F. J. M., van Os, J., & Drukker, M. (2021). Preschool communication: Early identification of concerns about preschool language development and social participation. *Frontiers in Public Health*, 8, 546536. https://doi.org/10.3389/fpubh.2020.546536

Drescher, J., Schwartz, A., Casoy, F., McIntosh, C. A., Hurley, B., Ashley, K., Barber, M., Goldenberg, D., Herbert, S. E., Lothwell, L. E., Mattson, M. R., McAfee, S. G., Pula, J., Rosario, V., & Tompkins, D. A. (2016). The growing regulation of conversion therapy. *Journal of Medical Regulation*, *102*(2), 7. https://doi.org/10.30770/2572-1852-102.2.7

Eaton, J. (2018). *A guide to mental health issues in girls and young women on the autism spectrum: Diagnosis, intervention, and family support*. Jessica Kingsley.

Ecker, B., Ticic, R., & Hulley, L. (2024). The Transformational psychotherapy of emotional unlearning. In B. Ecker, R. Ticic, and L. Hulley (Eds.), *Unlocking the emotional brain* (pp. 44–78). Routledge.

Epston, D. (1994). Extending the conversation. *Family Therapy Networker Nov/Dec.*

Erikson, E. (1959). *Identity and the life cycle*. International Universities Press.

Feldman, M., Hamsho, N., Blacher, J., Carter, A. S., & Eisenhower, A. (2022). Predicting peer acceptance and peer rejection for autistic children. *Psychology in the Schools*, *59*(11), 2159–2182. https://doi.org/10.1002/PITS.22739

Felitti, V. J., Anda, R. F., Nordenberg, D., Williamson, D. F., Spitz, A. M., Edwards, V., Koss, M. P., & Marks, J. S. (1998). Relationship of childhood abuse and household dysfunction to many of the leading causes of death in adults: The adverse childhood experiences (ACE) study. *American Journal of Preventive Medicine, 14*(4), 245–258. https://doi.org/10.1016/S0749-3797(98)00017-8

Fernandez-Prieto, M., Moreira, C., Cruz, S., Campos, V., Martínez-Regueiro, R., Taboada, M., Carracedo, A., & Sampaio, A. (2021). Executive functioning: A mediator between sensory processing and behaviour in Autism Spectrum Disorder. *Journal of Autism and Developmental Disorders, 51*(6), 2091–2103. https://doi.org/10.1007/S10803-020-04648-4

Fife, S. T., Whiting, J. B., Bradford, K., & Davis, S. (2014). The therapeutic pyramid: A common factors synthesis of techniques, alliance, and way of being. *Journal of Marital and Family Therapy, 40*(1), 20–33.

Fink, E., Olthof, T., Goossens, F., van der Meijden, S., & Begeer, S. (2018). Bullying-related behaviour in adolescents with autism: Links with autism severity and emotional and behavioural problems. *Autism, 22*(6), 684–692. https://doi.org/10.1177/1362361316686760

Finlay, L. (2021). *The therapeutic use of self in counselling and psychotherapy*. Sage Publications.

Fisher, J. (2014). Putting the pieces together: 25 years of learning trauma treatment. *Psychotherapy Networker, 38*(3), 33–39.

Fisher, W. W., Greer, B. D., & Mitteer, D. R. (2023). Additional comments on the use of contingent electric skin shock. *Perspectives on Behavior Science, 46*(2), 339–348. https://doi.org/10.1007/S40614-023-00382-1

Fisher, W. W., Piazza, C. C., & Roane, H. S. (2021). *Handbook of applied behavior analysis*. 624.

Fogel, A. (1993). *Developing through relationships*. University of Chicago Press.

Fraser, J. S. (2018). *Unifying effective psychotherapies: Tracing the process of change*. American Psychological Association.

Fusar-Poli, P., de Pablo, G. S., de Micheli, A., Nieman, D. H., Correll, C. U., Kessing, L. V., Pfennig, A., Bechdolf, A., Borgwardt, S., Arango, C., & van Amelsvoort, T. (2020). What is good mental health? A scoping review. *European Neuropsychopharmacology, 31*, 33–46.

Gable, S. (2006). Approach and avoidance social motives and goals. *Journal of Personality, 74*(1), 175–222.

Ganesan, B., Al-Jumaily, A., Fong, K. N., Prasad, P., Meena, S. K., & Tong, R. K. Y. (2021). Impact of coronavirus disease 2019 (COVID-19) outbreak quarantine, isolation, and lockdown policies on mental health and suicide. *Frontiers in Psychiatry, 12*. www.frontiersin.org/journals/psychiatry/articles/10.3389/fpsyt.2021.565190/full#h4

Gaskin, G. E. (2021). *Relational savoring in mothers of children with autism spectrum disorders: An attachment-based intervention*.

Gehart, D. R. (2010). *Mastering competencies in family therapy: A practical approach to theories and clinical case documentation*. Brooks/Cole.

Godat, D., & Czerny, E. J. (2021). Communication today: Were Watzlawick & Co. wrong? *Journal of Solution Focused Practices, 5*(2).

Grandin, T. (2007). Autism from the inside. *Educational Leadership, 64*(5), 29.

Grandin, T., & Panek, R. (2014). *The autistic brain: Helping different kinds of minds succeed*. Mariner Books.

Grandin, T., & Scariano, M. M. (1986). *Emergence: Labeled autistic*. Arena Press.

Grassmann, H., Stupiggia, M., & Porges, S. W. (2023). The science of embodiment: Trauma, body, and relationship. *International Body Psychotherapy Journal*, *22*(1), 149.

Greenberg, L. S. (2004). Emotion–focused therapy. *Clinical Psychology & Psychotherapy: An International Journal of Theory & Practice*, *11*(1), 3–16.

Grosse, M., & Grawe, K. (2002). Bern Inventory of Treatment Goals: Part 1. Development and first application of a taxonomy of treatment goal themes. *Psychotherapy Research*, *12*(1), 79–99.

Gutstein, S. E. (2000). *Autism Aspergers, solving the relationship puzzle: A new developmental program that opens the door to lifelong social & emotional growth*. Future Horizons.

Gutstein, S. (2009). *The RDI book*. The Connections Center.

Hagerty, B. M. K., Lynch-Sauer, J., Patusky, K. L., Bouwsema, M., & Collier, P. (1992). Sense of belonging: A vital mental health concept. *Archives of Psychiatric Nursing*, *6*(3), 172–177.

Hajek, A., & König, H. H. (2021). Do lonely and socially isolated individuals think they die earlier? The link between loneliness, social isolation and expectations of longevity based on a nationally representative sample. *Psychogeriatrics: The Official Journal of the Japanese Psychogeriatric Society*, *21*(4), 571–576. https://doi.org/10.1111/PSYG.12707

Hall, J. P., Batza, K., Streed, C. G., Boyd, B. A., & Kurth, N. K. (2020). Health disparities among sexual and gender minorities with autism spectrum disorder. *Journal of Autism and Developmental Disorders*, *50*(8), 3071–3077.

Hallmayer, J., Cleveland, S., Torres, A., Phillips, J., Cohen, B., Torigoe, T., Miller, J., Fedele, A., Collins, J., Smith, K., Lotspeich, L., Croen, L. A., Ozonoff, S., Lajonchere, C., Grether, J. K., Risch, N., Cleveland, M., & Cohen, M. (2011). Genetic heritability and shared environmental factors among twin pairs with autism HHS public access. *Archives of General Psychiatry*, *68*(11), 1095–1102. https://doi.org/10.1001/archgenpsychiatry.2011.76

Harrop, C., Amsbary, J., Towner-Wright, S., Reichow, B., & Boyd, B. A. (2019). That's what I like: The use of circumscribed interests within interventions for individuals with autism spectrum disorder. A systematic review. *Research in Autism Spectrum Disorders*, *57*, 63–86. https://doi.org/10.1016/J.RASD.2018.09.008

Hartman, L. M., Farahani, M., Moore, A., Manzoor, A., & Hartman, B. L. (2023). Organizational benefits of neurodiversity: Preliminary findings on autism and the bystander effect. *Autism Research*, *16*(10), 1989–2001. https://doi.org/10.1002/AUR.3012

Hatcher, R. L. (2021). Responsiveness, the relationship, and the working alliance in psychotherapy. In J. C. Watson & H. Wiseman (Eds.), *The responsive psychotherapist: Attuning to clients in the moment* (pp. 37–58). American Psychological Association.

Hebron, J., Humphrey, N., & Oldfield, J. (2015). Vulnerability to bullying of children with autism spectrum conditions in mainstream education: A multi-informant qualitative exploration. *Journal of Research in Special Educational Needs*, *15*(3), 185–193.

Henley, A. (2013). The necessity of belonging and other discoveries. *Creative Interventions with Children: A Transtheoretical Approach*, 2–12.

Henning, S., Buchheim, A., Beckh, K., Nolte, T., Brenk-Franz, K., Leichsenring, F., Strack, M., & Dinger, U. (2010). The influence of psychodynamically oriented therapists' attachment representations on outcome and alliance in inpatient psychotherapy. *Psychotherapy Research, 20*(2), 193–202.

Heselton, G. A., Rempel, G. R., & Nicholas, D. B. (2022). "Realizing the problem wasn't necessarily me": The meaning of childhood adversity and resilience in the lives of autistic adults. *International Journal of Qualitative Studies on Health and Well-Being, 17*(1). https://doi.org/10.1080/17482631.2022.2051237

Hewitson, J. (2018). *Autism: How to raise a happy autistic child*. Orion Spring.

Higgins, J. M., Arnold, S. R., Weise, J., Pellicano, E., & Trollor, J. N. (2021). Defining autistic burnout through experts by lived experience: Grounded Delphi method investigating# AutisticBurnout. *Autism, 25*(8), 2356–2369.

Hirvikoski, T., Mittendorfer-Rutz, E., Boman, M., Larsson, H., Lichtenstein, P., & Bölte, S. (2016). Premature mortality in autism spectrum disorder. *The British Journal of Psychiatry, 208*(3), 232–238.

Hobson, H., Cross, M., Jefferies, V., & Forster, M. (2022). What is the future of research on language and communication needs and mental health? A report by the Special Interest Research Group for Language, Communication and Mental Health. *Language and Communications SIRG*. (Updated December 12, 2022). In Mental Health Weekly Digest (page 614). https://doi.org/10.31234/OSF.IO/SDF8N

Hodgetts, S., Richards, K., & Park, E. (2018). Preparing for the future: Multi-stakeholder perspectives on autonomous goal setting for adolescents with autism spectrum disorders. *Disability and Rehabilitation, 40*(20), 2372–2379.

Holliday-Willey, L. (1999). *Pretending to be normal: Living with Asperger's syndrome*. Jessica Kingsley.

Hoover, D. W., & Kaufman, J. (2018). Adverse childhood experiences in children with autism spectrum disorder. *Current Opinion in Psychiatry, 31*(2), 128–132.

Horvath, A. O., & Luborsky, L. (1993). The role of the therapeutic alliance in psychotherapy. *Journal of Consulting and Clinical Psychology, 61*(4), 561–573.

Hours, C., Recasens, C., & Baleyte, J.-M. (2022). ASD and ADHD comorbidity: What are we talking about? *Frontiers in Psychiatry, 13*. https://doi.org/10.3389/FPSYT.2022.837424

Hughes, D. A. (1997). *Facilitating developmental attachment: The road to emotional recovery and behavioral change in foster and adopted children*. Jason Aronson.

Hughes, D. A. (2006). *Building the bonds of attachment: Awakening love in deeply troubled children*. Jason Aronson.

Hughes, D. A., & Baylin, J. (2012). *Brain-based parenting: The neuroscience of caregiving for healthy attachment*. WW Norton & Company.

Hughes, D. A., Golding, K. S., & Hudson, J. (2019). *Healing relational trauma with attachment-focused interventions: Dyadic developmental psychotherapy with children and families*. WW Norton & Company.

Hughes, K., Bellis, M. A., Hardcastle, K. A., Sethi, D., Butchart, A., Mikton, C., Jones, L., & Dunne, M. P. (2017). The effect of multiple adverse childhood experiences on health: A systematic review and meta-analysis. *The Lancet Public Health, 2*(8), 356–366.

Hull, L., Petrides, K. V., Allison, C., Smith, P., Baron-Cohen, S., Lai, M. C., & Mandy, W. (2017). "Putting on my best normal": Social camouflaging in adults with autism spectrum conditions. *Journal of Autism and Developmental Disorders*, *47*(8), 2519–2534. https://doi.org/10.1007/S10803-017-3166-5/TABLES/2

Husk, S. A. (2022). Cutting the IDEA's Gordian Knot: Accepting entanglements of disability and self and embracing a" best interests" approach to disciplining students with disabilities. *Journal of Laws & Educaction*, *51*, 86–143.

Ilyka, D., Johnson, M. H., & Lloyd-Fox, S. (2021). Infant social interactions and brain development: A systematic review. *Neuroscience and Biobehavioral Reviews*, *130*, 448–469.

Imel, Z. E., & Wampold, B. E. (2008). The Importance of treatment and the science of common factors in psychotherapy. In S. D. Brown & R. W. Lent (Eds.), *Handbook of counseling psychology* (4th ed., pp. 249–266). John Wiley & Sons.

Jackson-Perry, D., Rosqvist, H. B., Annable, J. L., & Kourti, M. (2020). Sensory strangers: Travels in normate sensory worlds. In *Neurodiversity studies* (pp. 125–149). Routledge.

James, I. (2005). *Asperger's syndrome and high achievement: Some very remarkable people*. Jessica Kingsley Publishers.

Jones, S. C., Gordon, C. S., Akram, M., Murphy, N., & Sharkie, F. (2022). Inclusion, exclusion and isolation of autistic people: Community attitudes and autistic people's experiences. *Journal of Autism and Developmental Disorders*, *52*(3), 1131–1142. https://doi.org/10.1007/S10803-021-04998-7/METRICS

Jones-Smith, E. (2013). *Strengths-based therapy: Connecting theory, practice and skills*. Sage Publications.

Karakaş, N. M., & Dağlı, F. Ş. (2019). The importance of attachment in infant and influencing factors. *Turkish Archives of Pediatrics*, *54*(2), 76–81.

Karatekin, C., & Hill, M. (2019). Expanding the original definition of Adverse Childhood Experiences (ACEs). *Journal of Child & Adolescent Trauma*, *12*(3), 289. https://doi.org/10.1007/S40653-018-0237-5

Kayrouz, R., & Hansen, S. (2020). I don't believe in miracles: Using the ecological validity model to adapt the miracle question to match the client's cultural preferences and characteristics. *Professional Psychology: Research and Practice*, *51*(3), 223.

Kazdin, A. E. (2013). *Behavior modification in applied settings* (7th ed.). Wadsworth/Thomson.

Kerns, C. M., & Kendall, P. C. (2012). The presentation and classification of anxiety in autism spectrum disorder. *Clinical Psychology: Science and Practice*, *19*(4), 323.

Kilroy, E., Aziz-Zadeh, L., & Cermak, S. (2019). Ayres theories of autism and sensory integration revisited: What contemporary neuroscience has to say. *Brain Sciences*, *9*(3), 68–88.

Klin, A., Danovitch, J. H., Merz, A. B., & Volkmar, F. R. (2007). Circumscribed interests in higher functioning individuals with autism spectrum disorders: An exploratory study. *Research and Practice for Persons with Severe Disabilities*, *32*(2), 89–100. https://doi.org/10.2511/RPSD.32.2.89

Kostouros, P. (2017). Shifting the effects of vicarious trauma and compassion fatigue Public presentation, Mount Royal University.

Kumar, S., Tansley-Hancock, O., Sedley, W., Winston, J. S., Callaghan, M. F., Allen, M., Cope, T. E., Gander, P. E., Bamiou, D. E., & Griffiths, T. D. (2017). The brain basis for misophonia. *Current Biology*, *27*(4), 527–533. https://doi.org/10.1016/J.CUB.2016.12.048

Kupferstein, H. (2018). Evidence of increased PTSD symptoms in autistics exposed to applied behavior analysis. *Advances in Autism*, *4*(1), 19–29. https://doi.org/10.1108/AIA-08-2017-0016

Lambert, N. M., Stillman, T. F., Hicks, J. A., Kamble, S., Baumeister, R. F., & Fincham, F. D. (2013). To belong is to matter. *Personality and Social Psychology Bulletin*, *39*(11), 1418–1427. https://doi.org/10.1177/0146167213499186

Lapakko, D. (2007). Communication is 93% nonverbal: An urban legend proliferates. *Communication and Theater Association of Minnesota Journal*, *34*(1), 7–19.

Lating, J. M., Barnett, J. E., & Horowitz, M. (2009). Increasing advocacy awareness within professional psychology training programs: The 2005 National Council of Schools and Programs of Professional Psychology Self-Study. *Training and Education in Professional Psychology*, *3*(2), 106.

Layle, P. (2024). *But everyone feels this way: How an autism diagnosis saved my life.* Hachette Go.

Leaf, J., Cihon, J., Ferguson, J., & Weiss, M. (2022). *Handbook of applied behavior analysis intervention for autism: Integrating research into practice – Autism and child psychopathology series: Vol. eBook.* https://link.springer.com/content/pdf/10.1007/978-3-030-96478-8.pdf

Leitner, Y. (2014). The co-occurrence of autism and attention deficit hyperactivity disorder in children–what do we know? *Frontiers in Human Neuroscience*, *8*, 268.

Levine, K. (2016). Replays: A therapeutic approach for children with autism spectrum disorder. In A. A. Drewes & C. E. Schaefer (Eds.), *Play therapy in middle childhood* (pp. 275–290). American Psychological Association.

Levine, P. A., Blakeslee, A., & Sylvae, J. (2018). Reintegrating fragmentation of the primitive self: Discussion of "somatic experiencing." *Psychoanalytic Dialogues*, *28*(5), 620–628.

Levy, K. N., & Johnson, B. N. (2019). Attachment and psychotherapy: Implications from empirical research. *Canadian Psychology/Psychologie Canadienne*, *60*(3), 178.

Lipinski, S., Boegl, K., Blanke, E. S., Suenkel, U., & Dziobek, I. (2022). A blind spot in mental healthcare? Psychotherapists lack education and expertise for the support of adults on the autism spectrum. *Autism*, *26*(6), 1509–1521.

Liu, S. (2019). Autism spectrum disorder. *Integration*, *804*, 754–0000.

Machingura, T., & Lloyd, C. (2017). Sensory approaches in mental health: Contemporary occupation-based practice or a redundant medical approach? *International Journal of Therapy and Rehabilitation*, *24*(5), 189. https://doi.org/10.12968/IJTR.2017.24.9.373

Maenner, M. J., Warren, Z., Williams, A. R., & et al. (2023). Prevalence and Characteristics of Autism Spectrum Disorder among children aged 8 years — autism and developmental disabilities monitoring network, 11 sites, United States, 2020. *MMWR Surveillance Summaries: 2023*, *72*(SS-2), 1–14.

Mahjoob, M., Paul, T., Carbone, J., Bokadia, H., Cardy, R. E., Kassam, S., Anagnostou, E., Andrade, B. F., Penner, M., & Kushki, A. (2023). Predictors of health-related quality of life in neurodivergent children: A systematic review. *Clinical Child and Family Psychology Review, 27*(1), 91–129. https://doi.org/10.1007/S10567-023-00462-3

Main, M. (1996). Introduction to the special section on attachment and psychopathology: 2. Overview of the field of attachment. *Journal of Consulting and Clinical Psychology, 64*(2), 237–243. https://doi.org/10.1037/0022-006X.64.2.237

Mallinckrodt, B. (2000). Attachment, social competencies, social support, and interpersonal process in psychotherapy. *Psychotherapy Research, 10*(3), 239–266.

Malloch, S., & Trevarthen, C. (2009). *Communicative musicality.* Oxford University Press.

Martin, D. J., Garske, J. P., & Davis, M. K. (2000). Relation of the therapeutic alliance with outcome and other variables: A meta-analytic review. *Journal of Consulting and Clinical Psychology, 68*(3), 438–450.

Masataka, N. (2017). Implications of the idea of neurodiversity for understanding the origins of developmental disorders. *Physics of Life Reviews, 20*, 85–108.

Maslow, A. H. (1954). *Motivation and personality.* Harper and Row.

Maté, G. (2011). *When the body says no: The cost of hidden stress.* Vintage Canada.

Mathur, S. K. (2021). *Understanding the lived experiences of autistic adults.* Chapman University.

Mazurek, M. O., Sadikova, E., Cheak-Zamora, N., Hardin, A., Sohl, K., & Malow, B. A. (2023). Health care needs, experiences, and perspectives of autistic adults. *Autism in Adulthood, 5*(1), 51–62.

McGreevy, S., & Boland, P. (2020). Sensory-based interventions with adult and adolescent trauma survivors: An integrative review of the occupational therapy literature. *Irish Journal of Occupational Therapy, 48*(1), 31–54. https://doi.org/10.1108/IJOT-10-2019-0014

McNamee, S. (2009). Postmodern psychotherapeutic ethics: Relational responsibility in practice. *Human Systems: The Journal of Therapy, Consultation & Training, 20*(1), 57–71.

Mehrabian, A. (1972). *Nonverbal communication* (1st ed.). Routledge.

Mehrabian, A., & Ferris, S. R. (1967). Inference of attitudes from nonverbal communication in two channels. *Journal of Consulting Psychology, 31*(3), 248–252.

Mehrabian, A., & Wiener, M. (1967). Decoding of inconsistent communications. *Journal of Personality and Social Psychology, 6*(1), 109–114.

Menesini, E., & Salmivalli, C. (2017). Bullying in schools: The state of knowledge and effective interventions. *Psychology, Health & Medicine, 22*, 240–253. https://doi.org/10.1080/13548506.2017.1279740

Milton, D. E. (2012). On the ontological status of autism: The 'double empathy problem.' *Disability & Society, 27*(6), 883–887.

Minshawi, N. F., Hurwitz, S., Fodstad, J. C., Biebl, S., Morriss, D. H., & Mcdougle, C. J. (2014). The association between self-injurious behaviors and autism spectrum disorders. *Psychology Research and Behavior Management, 7*, 125–136. https://doi.org/10.2147/PRBM.S44635

Moran, H. (2010). Clinical observations of the differences between children on the autism spectrum and those with attachment problems: The Coventry Grid. *Good Autism Practice (GAP), 11*(2), 46–59.

Morgan, H. (2019). Connections between sensory sensitivities in autism; The importance of sensory friendly environments for accessibility and increased quality of life for the neurodivergent autistic minority. *PSU McNair Scholars Online Journal*, *13*(1), 1.

Moseley, R. L., Gregory, N. J., Smith, P., Allison, C., & Baron-Cohen, S. J. M. A. (2019). A 'choice', an 'addiction', a way 'out of the lost': Exploring self-injury in autistic people without intellectual disability. *Molecular Autism, 10*, 1–23.

Muris, P., & Ollendick, T. H. (2021). Selective mutism and its relations to social anxiety disorder and autism spectrum disorder. *Clinical Child and Family Psychology Review*, *24*(2), 294–325.

Neff, M. A. (2024). *Self-care for autistic people*. Simon & Schuster.

Nerenberg, J. (2020). *Divergent mind: Thriving in a world that wasn't designed for you*. HarperOne.

Nesin-Perna, S. (2023). *The interaction of mental health and executive function among neurodiverse University students* [Doctoral Dissertation]. University of Massachusetts Lowell.

Ofner, M., Coles, A., Decou, M. L., Do, M., Bienek, A., Snider, J., & Ugnat, A. (2018). *Autism spectrum disorder among children and youth in Canada 2018*. Public Health Agency of Canada.

Oliphant, R. Y., Smith, E. M., & Grahame, V. (2020). What is the prevalence of self-harming and suicidal behaviour in under 18s with ASD, with or without an intellectual disability? *Journal of Autism and Developmental Disorders, 50*(10), 3510–3524.

Olweus, D. (2013). School bullying: Development and some important challenges. *Annual Review of Clinical Psychology, 9*, 751–780. https://doi.org/10.1146/ANNU REV-CLINPSY-050212-185516

O'Nions, E., Petersen, I., Buckman, J. E. J., Charlton, R., Cooper, C., & Corbett, A. (2023). Autism in England: Assessing underdiagnosis in a population-based cohort study of prospectively collected primary care data. *The Lancet Regional Health – Europe, 29*, 100626.

Panagiotidi, M., Overton, P. G., & Stafford, T. (2019). Co-occurrence of ASD and ADHD traits in an adult population. *Journal of Attention Disorders, 23*(12), 1407–1415.

Parham, L. D., & Crickmore, D. (2022). *Expanding sensory awareness. Intellectual disabilities-E-book: Toward inclusion* (Vol. 231). Elsevier Health Sciences.

Parmar, K. R., Porter, C. S., Dickinson, C. M., Pelham, J., Baimbridge, P., & Gowen, E. (2021). Visual sensory experiences from the viewpoint of autistic adults. *Frontiers in Psychology, 12*, 633037.

Parsons, C. E., Young, K. S., Murray, L., Stein, A., & Kringelbach, M. L. (2010). The functional neuroanatomy of the evolving parent-infant relationship. *Progress in Neurobiology, 91*, 220–241. https://doi.org/10.1016/j.pneurobio.2010.03.001

Patel, V., Saxena, S., Lund, C., Thornicroft, G., Baingana, F., Bolton, P., Chisholm, D., Collins, P. Y., Cooper, J. L., Eaton, J., & Herrman, H. (2018). The Lancet Commission on global mental health and sustainable development. *The Lancet, 392*(10157), 1553–1598.

Paxton, K., & Estay, I. A. (2007). *Counselling people on the autism spectrum: A practical manual*. Jessica Kingsley.

Pearson, A., & Rose, K. (2021). A conceptual analysis of autistic masking: Understanding the narrative of stigma and the illusion of choice. *Autism in Adulthood: Challenges and Management, 3*(1), 52. https://doi.org/10.1089/AUT.2020.0043

Pearson, A., Rose, K., & Rees, J. (2023). 'I felt like I deserved it because I was autistic': Understanding the impact of interpersonal victimisation in the lives of autistic people. *Autism, 27*(2), 500–511.

Perry, B. D. (2007). Stress, trauma and post-traumatic stress disorders in children. *The Child Trauma Academy, 17*, 42–57.

Perry, B. D. (2014). The neurosequential model of therapeutics in young children. In K. Brandt, B. D. Perry, S. Seligman, & E. Tronick (Eds.), *Infant and early childhood mental health* (pp. 21–47). American Psychiatric Press.

Perry, B. D., & Winfrey, O. (2021). *What happened to you?: Conversations on trauma, resilience, and healing.* Flatiron Books: An Oprah Book.

Phillips, A. (2010). *On balance.* Farrar, Straus and Giroux.

Phillips, S., & Melim, D. (2020). *Belonging: A relationship-based approach for trauma-informed education.* Rowman & Littlefield Publishers.

Phung, J., Penner, M., Pirlot, C., & Welch, C. (2021). What I wish you knew: Insights on burnout, inertia, meltdown, and shutdown from autistic youth. *Frontiers in Psychology, 12*, 741421.

Pinto, R. Z., Ferreira, M. L., Oliveira, V. C., Franco, M. R., Adams, R., Maher, C. G., & Ferreira, P. H. (2012). Patient-centred communication is associated with positive therapeutic alliance: A systematic review. *Journal of Physiotherapy, 58*(2), 77–87. https://doi.org/10.1016/S1836-9553(12)70087-5

Pittman, C. M., & Karle, E. M. (2015). *Rewiring the anxious brain. How to use the neuroscience of fear to end anxiety, panic and worry.* New Harbinger Publications.

Porges, S. W., & Dana, D. (2018). *Clinical applications of the polyvagal theory: The emergence of polyvagal-informed therapies (Norton series on interpersonal neurobiology).* WW Norton & Company.

Porter, C., Baimbridge, P., & Pelham, J. (2021). Visual sensory experiences from the viewpoint of autistic adults. *Frontiers in Psychology, 12*, 633037. https://doi.org/10.3389/fpsyg.2021.633037

Predescu, E., Sipos, R., Costescu, C. A., Ciocan, A., & Rus, D. I. (2020). Executive functions and emotion regulation in attention-deficit/hyperactivity disorder and borderline intellectual disability. *Journal of Clinical Medicine, 9*(4), 986. https://doi.org/10.3390/JCM9040986

Price. D. (2022). *Unmasking autism: Discovering the new faces of neurodiversity.* Harmony.

Prochaska, J. O., & DiClemente, C. (1982). Trans-theoretical therapy-toward a more integrative model of change. *Psychotherapy: Theory, Research & Practice, 19*(3), 276–288. https://doi.org/10.1037/h0088437

Prochaska, J. O., & Norcross, J. C. (2001). Stages of change. *Psychotherapy, 38*(4), 443–448. https://doi.org/10.1037/0033-3204.38.4.443

Public Health Agency of Canada. (2022). *Autism spectrum disorder: Highlights from the 2019 Canadian health survey on children and youth.*

Purkey, E., Patel, R., & Phillips, S. P. (2018). Trauma-informed care: Better care for everyone. *Canadian Family Physician, 64*(3), 170–172.

Radulski, E. M. (2022). Conceptualising autistic masking, camouflaging, and neurotypical privilege: Towards a minority group model of neurodiversity. *Human Development, 66*(2), 113–127.

Randell, E., Wright, M., Milosevic, S., Gillespie, D., Brookes-Howell, L., Busse-Morris, M., Hastings, R., Maboshe, W., Williams-Thomas, R., Mills, L., Romeo, R., Yaziji, N., McKigney, A. M., Ahuja, A., Warren, G., Glarou, E., Delport, S., & McNamara, R. (2022). Sensory integration therapy for children with autism and sensory processing difficulties: The SenITA RCT. *Health Technology Assessment, 26*(29), 2. https://doi.org/10.3310/TQGE0020

Raymaker, D. M., Teo, A. R., Steckler, N. A., Lentz, B., Scharer, M., Delos Santos, A., Kapp, S. K., Hunter, M., Joyce, A., & Nicolaidis, C. (2020). "Having all of your internal resources exhausted beyond measure and being left with no clean-up crew": Defining autistic burnout. *Autism in Adulthood: Challenges and Management, 2*(2), 132–143. https://doi.org/10.1089/AUT.2019.0079

Rees, C. (2007). Childhood attachment. *British Journal of General Practice, 57*(544), 920–922.

Reiersen, A. M., & Todd, R. D. (2008). Co-occurrence of ADHD and autism spectrum disorders: Phenomenology and treatment. *Expert Review of Neurotherapeutics, 8*(4), 657–669. https://doi.org/10.1586/14737175.8.4.657

Rizou, E., & Giannouli, V. (2020). An exploration of the experience of trainee integrative psychotherapists on therapeutic alliance in the light of their attachment style. *Health Psychology Research, 8*(3), 153–166.

Robledo, J. A., & Donnellan, A. (2008). Properties of supportive relationships from the perspective of academically successful individuals with autism. *Intellectual and Developmental Disabilities, 46*(4), 299–310.

Rogers, C. R. (1949). The attitude and orientation of the counselor in client-centered therapy. *Journal of Consulting Psychology, 13*(2), 82–94.

Rogers, C. R. (1959). A theory of therapy, personality, and interpersonal relationships as developed in the client-centered framework. In S. Koch (Ed.), *Psychology: A study of a science: Vol. 3.* McGraw Hill.

Rojas, M., Méndez, A., & Watkins-Fassler, K. (2023). The hierarchy of needs empirical examination of Maslow's theory and lessons for development. *World Development, 165.* https://doi.org/10.1016/j.worlddev.2023.106185

Rong, Y., Yang, C. J., Jin, Y., & Wang, Y. (2021). Prevalence of attention-deficit/hyperactivity disorder in individuals with autism spectrum disorder: A meta-analysis. *Research in Autism Spectrum Disorders, 83*(3), 101759. https://doi.org/10.1016/J.RASD.2021.101759

Rosenzweig, S. (1936). Some implicit common factors in diverse methods of psychotherapy. *American Journal of Orthopsychiatry, 6*(3), 412–415. https://doi.org/10.1111/J.1939-0025.1936.TB05248.X

Rowland, D. (2020). Redefining autism. *Journal of Neurology, Psychiatry and Brain Research (JNPBR), 02,* 148. https://doi.org/10.37722/JNPABR.20202

Rushton, A., Monck, E., Leese, M., McCrone, P., & Sharac, J. (2010). Enhancing adoptive parenting: A randomized controlled trial. *Clinical Child Psychology and Psychiatry, 15*(4), 529–542.

Russell, A. J., Jassi, A., Fullana, M. A., Mack, H., Johnston, K., Heyman, I., Murphy, D. G., & Mataix-Cols, D. (2013). Cognitive behavior therapy for comorbid obsessive-compulsive disorder in high-functioning autism spectrum disorders: A randomized controlled trial. *Depression and Anxiety, 30*(8), 697–708.

Russell, G., Kapp, S. K., Elliott, D., Elphick, C., Gwernan-Jones, R., & Owens, C. (2019). Mapping the autistic advantage from the accounts of adults diagnosed with autism: A qualitative study. *Autism in Adulthood, 1*(2), 124. https://doi.org/10.1089/AUT.2018.0035

Saakvitne, K. W., & Pearlman, L. A. (1996). *Transforming the pain: A workbook on vicarious traumatization.* WW Norton & Co.

Sandoval-Norton, A. H., & Shkedy, G. (2019). How much compliance is too much compliance: Is long-term ABA therapy abuse? *Cogent Psychology, 6*(1). https://doi.org/10.1080/23311908.2019.1641258

Saunders, P. (2018). Neurodivergent rhetorics: Examining competing discourses of autism advocacy in the public sphere. *Journal of Literary & Cultural Disability Studies, Liverpool University Press, 12*(1), 1–17.

Schauenburg, H., Buchheim, A., Beckh, K., Nolte, T., Brenk-Franz, K., Leichsenring, F., Strack, M., & Dinger, U. (2010). The influence of psychodynamically oriented therapists' attachment representations on outcome and alliance in inpatient psychotherapy. *Psychotherapy Research, 20*(2), 193–202.

Schmeck, K., Schlüter-Müller, S., Foelsch, P. A., & Doering, S. (2013). The role of identity in the DSM-5 classification of personality disorders. *Child and Adolescent Psychiatry and Mental Health, 7*, 1–11.

Sedgewick, F., Hull, L., & Ellis, H. (2021). *Autism and masking: How and why people do it, and the impact it can have.* Jessica Kingsley Publishers.

Segers, M., & Rawana, J. (2014). What do we know about suicidality in autism spectrum disorders? A systematic review. *Autism Research, 7*(4), 507–521.

Shanker, S. (2010). Self-Regulation: Calm, alert, and learning. *Education Canada, 50*(3), 4–7.

Shaw, S. C., Carravallah, L., Johnson, M., O'Sullivan, J., Chown, N., Neilson, S., & Doherty, M. (2023). Barriers to healthcare and a 'triple empathy problem' may lead to adverse outcomes for autistic adults: A qualitative study. *Autism: the international journal of research and practice, 13623613231205629. Advance online publication.* https://doi.org/10.1177/13623613231205629.

Sheppard, E., Webb, S., & Wilkinson, H. (2023). Mindreading beliefs in same-and cross-neurotype interactions. *Autism, 18*, 13623613231211456.

Simone, R. (2010a). *Asperger's on the job: Must-have advice for people with Asperger's or high functioning autism and their employers, educators, and advocates.* Future Horizins.

Simone, R. (2010b). *Aspergirls: Empowering females with Asperger syndrome.* Jessica Kingsley Publishers.

Skinner, B. F. (1953). *Science and human behavior.* Macmillan.

Snodgrass, J. G., Lacy, M. G., & Upadhyay, C. (2017). Developing culturally sensitive affect scales for global mental health research and practice: Emotional balance, not named syndromes, in Indian Adivasi subjective well-being. *Social Science & Medicine, 187*, 174–183.

Solden, S., & Frank, M. (2019). *A radical guide for women with ADHD: Embrace neurodiversity, live boldly and break through barriers.* New Harbinger.

Specht, M. W., Woods, D. W., Nicotra, C. M., Kelly, L. M., Ricketts, E. J., Conelea, C. A., Grados, M. A., Ostrander, R. S., & Walkup, J. T. (2013). Effects of tic suppression: Ability to suppress, rebound, negative reinforcement, and habituation to the premonitory urge. *Behaviour Research and Therapy, 51*(1), 24–30. https://doi.org/10.1016/J.BRAT.2012.09.009

Sperry, L. (2005a). Case conceptualization: A strategy for incorporating individual, couple and family dynamics in the treatment process. *American Journal of Family Therapy, 33*, 353–364.

Sperry, L. (2005b). Case conceptualizations: The missing link between theory and practice. *The Family Journal, 13*(1), 71–76. https://doi.org/10.1177/1066480704270104

Staddon, J. E. R., & Cerutti, D. T. (2003). Operant conditioning. *Annual Review of Psychology, 54*(1), 115–144.

Stockman, J. (2023). *Notes for neuro navigators: The allies' quick-start guide to championing neurodivergent brains*. Jessica Kingsley Publishers.

Strunz, R. M. (2018). Common factors of a transtheoretical model of Autism Spectrum Disorder-informed psychotherapy. *Canadian Journal of Counselling and Psychotherapy, 52*(3).

Suchy, Y. (2009). Executive functioning: Overview, assessment, and research issues for non-neuropsychologists. *Annals of Behavioral Medicine: A Publication of the Society of Behavioral Medicine, 37*(2), 106–116. https://doi.org/10.1007/S12160-009-9097-4

Sue, D. W. (2010a). *Microaggressions and marginality: Manifestation, dynamics, and impact* (D. W. Sue, Ed.). John Wiley & Sons.

Sue, D. W. (2010b). *Microaggressions in everyday life: Race, gender, and sexual orientation*. John Wiley & Sons, Inc.

Sue, D. W., Capodilupo, C. M., Torino, G. C., Bucceri, J. M., Holder, A. M. B., Nadal, K. L., & Esquilin, M. (2007). Racial microaggressions in everyday life: Implications for clinical practice. *American Psychologist, 62*(4), 271–286.

Sue, D. W., & Spanierman, L. (2020). *Microaggressions in everyday life*. John Wiley & Sons.

Sussman, M. (2007). *A curious calling: Unconscious motivations for practicing psychotherapy* (2nd ed.). Jason Aronson.

Sutton, D., Wilson, M., van Kessel, K., & Vanderpyl, J. (2013). Optimizing arousal to manage aggression: A pilot study of sensory modulation. *International Journal of Mental Health Nursing, 22*(6), 500–511. https://doi.org/10.1111/INM.12010

Sweeney, A., Filson, B., Kennedy, A., Collinson, L., & Gillard, S. (2018). A paradigm shift: Relationships in trauma-informed mental health services. *BJPsych Advances, 24*(5), 319. https://doi.org/10.1192/BJA.2018.29

Sylvester, E., & Scherer, K. (2022). *Relationship-based treatment of children and their parents: An integrative guide to neurobiology, attachment, regulation, and discipline (IPNB)*. WW Norton and Company.

Tang, N., Bensman, L., & Hatfield, E. (2013). Culture and sexual self-disclosure in intimate relationships. *Interpersona: An International Journal on Personal Relationships, 7*(2), 227–245.

Teague, S. J., Gray, K. M., Tonge, B. J., & Newman, L. K. (2017). Attachment in children with autism spectrum disorder: A systematic review. *Research in Autism Spectrum Disorders, 35*, 35–50.

Timulak, L., & Keogh, D. (2017). The client's perspective on (experiences of) psycho-therapy: A practice friendly review. *Journal of Clinical Psychology, 73*(11), 1556–1567. https://doi.org/10.1002/JCLP.22532

Toporek, R. L., Gerstein, L., Fouad, N., Roysircar, G., & Israel, T. (2005). *Handbook for social justice in counseling psychology: Leadership, vision, and action.* Sage Publications.

Tourjman, V., Louis-Nascan, G., Ahmed, G., DuBow, A., Côté, H., Daly, N., & Sadek, J. (2022). Psychosocial interventions for attention deficit/hyperactivity disorder: A sys-tematic review and Meta-analysis by the CADDRA guidelines Work GROUP. *Brain Sciences, 12*(8), 1023.

Trevisan, D. A., Roberts, N., Lin, C., & Birmingham, E. (2017). How do adults and teens with self-declared Autism Spectrum Disorder experience eye contact? A qualitative analysis of first-hand accounts. *PLoS ONE, 12*(11), e0188446. https://doi.org/10.1371/journal.pone.0188446, www.ncbi.nlm.nih.gov/pmc/articles/PMC5705114.

Twyman, K. A., Saylor, C. F., Saia, D., Macias, M. M., Taylor, L. A., & Spratt, E. (2010). Bullying and ostracism experiences in children with special health care needs. *Journal of Developmental and Behavioral Pediatrics, 31*(1), 1–8. https://doi.org/10.1097/DBP.0B013E3181C828C8

Tyler, T. A. (2012). The limbic model of systemic trauma. *Journal of Social Work Practice, 26*(1), 125–138.

Ulmer-Yaniv, A., Waidergoren, S., Shaked, A., Salomon, R., & Feldman, R. (2022). Neural representation of the parent–child attachment from infancy to adulthood. *Social Cognitive and Affective Neuroscience, 17*(7), 609–624.

Umagami, K., Remington, A., Lloyd-Evans, B., Davies, J., & Crane, L. (2022). Loneliness in autistic adults: A systematic review. *Autism, 26*(8), 2117–2135. https://doi.org/10.1177/13623613221077721/ASSET/IMAGES/LARGE/10.1177_13623613221077721-FIG1.JPEG

Vaillant, G. E. (2012). Positive mental health: Is there a cross-cultural definition? *World Psychiatry, 11*(2), 93–99.

van der Kolk, B. A. (2003). *Psychological trauma.* American Psychiatric Pub.

van Roekel, E., Scholte, R. H. J., & Didden, R. (2010). Bullying among adolescents with Autism Spectrum Disorders: Prevalence and perception. *Journal of Autism and Developmental Disorders, 40*(1), 63. https://doi.org/10.1007/S10803-009-0832-2

Vanhee, G., Lemmens, G., & Verhofstadt, L. L. (2016). Relationship satisfaction: High need satisfaction or low need frustration? *Social Behavior and Personality: An International Journal, 44*(6), 923–930.

Vos, J. (2018). *Meaning in life: An evidence-based handbook for practitioners.* Bloomsbury Publishing.

Wampold, B. E. (2015). How important are the common factors in psychotherapy? An update. *World Psychiatry, 14*(3), 270. https://doi.org/10.1002/WPS.20238

Watzlawick, P., Bavelas, J. B., & Jackson, D. D. (2011). *Pragmatics of human commu-nication: A study of interactional patterns, pathologies and paradoxes.* WW Norton & Company.

Webster, A. A., & Garvis, S. (2017). The importance of critical life moments: An explora-tive study of successful women with autism spectrum disorder. *Autism, 21*(6), 670–677.

Wei, X., Yu, J. W., Shattuck, P., McCracken, N., & Blackorby, J. (2012). Science, technology, engineering, and mathematics (STEM) participation among college students with an autism spectrum disorder. *Journal of Autism and Developmental Disorders*, *43*, 1539.

Weiss, J. A. (2003). Self-injurious behaviours in autism: A literature review. *Journal on Developmental Disabilities*, *9*(2), 127–144.

White, M. (1994). Ritual of inclusion: An approach to extreme uncontrolled behaviour in children and young adolescents. *Journal of Child and Youth Care*, *9*, 51–51.

Williams, A. (2018). Autonomously autistic. *Canadian Journal of Disability Studies*, *7*(2), 60–82. https://doi.org/10.15353/CJDS.V7I2.423

Wilson, B., Beamish, W., Hay, S., & Attwood, T. (2014). Prompt dependency beyond childhood: Adults with Asperger's syndrome and intimate relationships. *Journal of Relationships Research*, *5*. https://doi.org/10.1017/JRR.2014.11

World Health Organization. (2004). *Promoting mental health: Concepts, emerging evidence, practice: Summary report*. World Health Organization.

World Health Organization. (2022a). *Mental health fact sheet*. United Nations.

World Health Organization. (2022b). *World mental health report: Transforming mental health for all*.

Wu, M. B., & Levitt, H. M. (2022). How to become a responsive therapist: A study of experiences of developing therapists. *Psychotherapy Research*, *32*(6), 763–777.

Yalom, I. D. (2002). *The gift of therapy: An open letter to a new generation of therapists and their patients*. HarperCollins.

Yuan, P., & Raz, N. (2014). Prefrontal cortex and executive functions in healthy adults: A meta-analysis of structural neuroimaging studies. *Neuroscience & Biobehavioral Reviews*, *42*, 180–192.

Zautra, A. J., Hall, J. S., Murray, K. E., & Resilience Solutions Group 1. (2008). Resilience: A new integrative approach to health and mental health research. *Health Psychology Review*, *2*(1), 41–64.

Zeanah, C. H., & Gleason, M. M. (2015). Annual research review: Attachment disorders in early childhood–clinical presentation, causes, correlates, and treatment. *Journal of Child Psychology and Psychiatry*, *56*(3), 207–222.

Index